THE FIDGET FACTOR

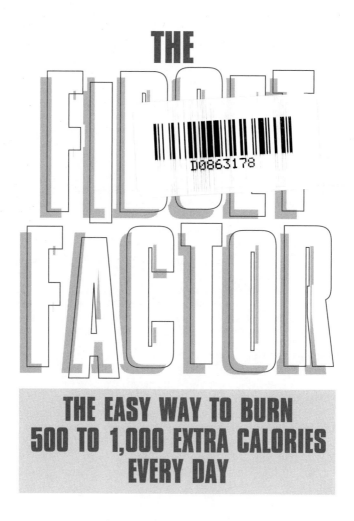

THE EASY WAY TO BURN 500 TO 1,000 EXTRA CALORIES EVERY DAY

Frank I. Katch and Victor L. Katch
with Gene Brown

A Stonesong Press Book

**Andrews McMeel
Publishing**
Kansas City

00 01 02 03 04 VHG 10 9 8 7 6 5 4 3 2 1

Library of Congress Cataloging-in-Publication Data
Katch, Frank I.
    The fidget factor : the easy way to burn up to 1000 extra calories every day / Frank Katch and Victor Katch, with Gene Brown.
        p. cm
    ISBN 0-7407-1009-5 (pbk.)
        1. Weight loss. 2. Exercise. I. Katch, Victor L. II. Brown, Gene. III. Title.

RM222.2 .K349 2000
613.7—dc21   00-35578

A Stonesong Press Book

ATTENTION: SCHOOLS AND BUSINESSES

Andrews McMeel books are available at quantity discounts with bulk purchase for educational, businesss, or sales promotional use. For information, please write to: Special Sales Department, Andrews McMeel Publishing, 4520 Main Street, Kansas City, Missouri 64111.

CONTENTS

PREFACE

One fact about our health in the early twenty-first century should make all Americans fidget. For the first time, over half our population is overweight. True, our life expectancy has increased, medical procedures repair injuries, and machinery helps us work. But most of us suffer from obesity. How we deal with being "stocky" is a serious problem, because weight gain encourages the crippling consequences of heart disease, diabetes, stroke, and psychological depression. For nearly 150 years we have been advised to balance our food intake with physical activity. Recently, we have spent millions of dollars on questionable diets and faddish exercise equipment. Still, Americans of all ages and social classes are putting on an unprecedented number of pounds. We know the very conveniences that comfort us—cars and escalators, for example—also lessen our need to exert ourselves. And as we accumulate more birthdays, we usually decrease the movement that can burn off some of the 1,900 pounds of food that an average adult consumes yearly.

Can we do anything to combat this frightening invasion of excess calories? Few of us can or should eat cabbage soup or "spot reduce" for long. What we all need are reasonable physical activities we can incorporate into our ordinary days. As experienced professors of exercise science and kinesiology, we respect the powerful truth: A healthy body burns the excess calories it does not need.

But rather than urging you to purchase some hunger-killing powder or coaxing you to train for a marathon, we share with you practical ways to balance calories by increasing daily physical activities. Who should be alarmed by weight gain? All of us. Who can profit from the following suggestions? Again, all of us, including children, partners, professionals, retired folk, and, yes, the authors ourselves. Help us to realize our dream of a healthy nation, one populated by fit people of all body types united by the same agenda: They burn unnecessary calories. So join us right now as we walk, lift, wiggle, jump, bend, shake, climb. Let's become fellow fidgeters!

Here's to a happy and healthy life.

FRANK I. KATCH
Professor of Exercise Science
University of Massachusetts
Amherst, Massachusetts

VICTOR L. KATCH
Professor of Kinesiology
University of Michigan
Ann Arbor, Michigan

CHAPTER 1

FIDGETING AS A FACTOR IN AN EFFECTIVE WEIGHT-CONTROL PLAN

BEING OVERWEIGHT CAN KILL YOU. IF EVER THERE WAS any doubt about it, a fourteen-year study by the American Cancer Society involving 1 million people, reported in *The New England Journal of Medicine* and headlined in every major paper in the country, showed that excess pounds can end your life early. In fact, scientists at the University of Texas Medical School recently reported that approximately 250,000 deaths each year in this country are related to physical inactivity.

What's more, the study showed the depressing effect of too much body fat on your life span independent of any other factor. Even if you strip away other factors such as smoking, high blood pressure, and too little cardiovascular exercise, being overweight puts you in harm's way—from the prime of your life right through to your later years.

If you're reading this book, you have most likely tried some combination of diet and exercise to deal with your excess weight. You may even have made some progress. But getting to where you want to be and staying there may always have seemed out of reach. If so, welcome to the club. More than half of adult Americans are like you.

There should be no surprise that the diet- and weight-control industry is a multibillion-dollar enterprise in this country and abroad, and it's growing.

Now here's the good news—great news, in fact. You've had an important, easy-to-use weapon in your war on body fat at your disposal all the time, waiting for you to use it. It's a weight-control technique that's conservative, scientific, as cheap as it comes, healthy, and, best of all, realistic. By the time you've finished reading about it, you'll have wondered, "Why didn't I think of that?"

YOU'RE ABOUT TO HAVE A MOVING EXPERIENCE

How would you like to burn several hundred calories a day beyond what you already burn? That's *several hundred calories* above and beyond what you already consume through your physical activity. Would you like it even more if these delightfully productive activities blended into what you do anyway in the course of a day—activities so undemanding and so unobtrusive that they don't require you to sacrifice any part of your busy schedule?

What if this convenient adjunct to a sensible diet and moderate exercise were enough to put you steadily over the top in meeting those weight-reduction goals that you never quite attain—say, to the tune of losing an extra pound or two every month, month after month, until you achieve your goal without working up a sweat?

Most important, what if it were something that required little effort on your part to *keep doing*, that wouldn't fall by the wayside because it was snowing and you couldn't get to the gym, or your child was sick and you had to forgo heavy workouts for five days, or you just got bored? What if it were simply there for you to access, on demand, wherever you were, whenever you wanted it?

You may not realize it yet, but you already have a handle on what this plan is all about. It's what your parents and teachers told you not to do when you were a kid: fidget.

IT'S ALL AROUND YOU

Fidgeting is like the wallpaper of life—almost always there but hardly noticed. If that seems far-fetched, just look around you.

Even if you're not a baseball fan, you've probably seen a pitcher standing on the mound, pulling at the visor of his cap, tugging on his pants belt, rubbing the ball, kicking the dirt out of his cleats, and then starting this routine all over again. Meanwhile, the coach at third base is pulling his ear, scratching the back of his head, putting one hand on his hip, and then tugging at *his* cap. What's eating these guys?

These grown men are fidgeting in front of thousands of people in the stands and possibly millions on television. If they were children, their mothers would probably tell them to cut it out. But they are grown-ups and their seemingly aimless movements have a purpose. The coach is sending a secret signal to the batter, telling him what do on the next pitch. And the pitcher is trying to relax and get into an effective, comfortable rhythm.

You don't have to be a baseball player to fidget. We probably all do it to some extent as adults and did it even more when we were children. Teachers often put their hands on their hips, scratch the back of their heads, and shift from one foot to the other when listening to a student respond to a lesson. Your colleagues at work may shift in their seats and put their hands on the back of their heads while you are delivering a report. And the clerk at the post office may fold and unfold his arms, move his hand to his chin, and tap a pencil while you explain that the package you've come to pick up *must* be there.

You may even know people who fidget to the point of distracting others with their nervous mannerisms. But *we* know of no one outside of sports who ever fidgeted with a conscious purpose—until recently.

Now it turns out that fidgeting, this most overlooked of human activities, can actually help you control and even lose weight! That's no wild claim from the likes of the patent medicine salesman. Nor is it some kind of a far-out, no-fault cure for excess pounds pushed on late-night cable TV by a company that would love to sell you its "fidget" seminar on a set of expensive videotapes.

This very useful function for what always seemed like an aimless waste of energy surfaced only at the beginning of 1998 as a result of an experiment at the world-famous Mayo Clinic. Under controlled conditions, doctors there determined that people who fidgeted were burning extra calories, just as they would if they were doing more formal exercises. They weren't burning off a huge amount. But for some people it added up to a few hundred calories a day—potentially as many as 800—and that would be enough to make a difference of a pound or so of body weight each week if one fidgeted regularly. If you've ever wanted to control your weight or lose some pounds, you can appreciate what that might mean over the course of several months or a year or more.

WHAT YOU CAN EXPECT

The Fidget Factor will tell you about the exciting implications of this significant discovery for your life. You will

BEEN DOIN' IT FOR YEARS

It's not unusual these days to discover that something you've been accustomed to doing all your life—such as fidgeting—suddenly has a useful, healthy purpose you knew nothing about. For example, would you have believed a few years ago that the common tomato, especially when cooked, contained substances that may well protect you against certain kinds of cancer? Who might have guessed that the joke your friend used to make about having a glass of red wine with dinner strictly for "medicinal" purposes was unintentionally more than a jest because it does appear to help protect against heart disease?

see that you don't have to be a nervous jervis to make fidgeting work for you, just more attentive to how much and how you move during the day. You'll see how the potential power of fidgeting fits in the context of the diet and more conventional exercise you've probably already tried. You're going to see how fidgeting and related moderate, informal exercising—embedded in your daily activities —can seriously contribute to your efforts to look and feel good.

The Fidget Factor will also show you *how* and *why* fidgeting works as a means of weight control, how you can easily learn to fidget if that's not something you do naturally, and how you can look at your environment with an eye toward finding easy opportunities to add these eminently useful and totally flexible activities to your daily routine so that after a while you'll hardly notice that you are *doing* anything.

The Fidget Factor will also describe 159 ways you can make use of fidgeting activities and low-level exercises to control your weight—enough possibilities to fit into anyone's lifestyle. We will tell you exactly how many calories you will be burning through every type of fidgeting and moderate exercise you could imagine, and you will be able to compare the amount of calories burned through these activities with the amount you would have burned by exercising more strenuously.

For example, if you run for forty-five minutes you'll burn around 500 calories. But if you fill the spare moments in your week with activities such as standing while talking on the phone, parking the car a little farther out in the lot, bouncing up and down on your toes while waiting on line—get the picture?—you can equal that calorie burn without the sweat.

The Fidget Factor does not promise pie in the sky (and not just because that, too, probably has too many calories). If you are clinically obese or substantially overweight, fidgeting will not change your life. Also, all the fidgeting in the world won't make much of a dent if you don't pay reasonable attention to how much and what kinds of food you eat, and it will probably fall short of the results you seek if you don't get at least some more rigorous exercise during the week.

We call it the *fidget factor* because it is a new and important element that can become part of your overall plan to stay fit and trim. It is not the entire solution but rather a component of your overall health plan that can finally spell the difference between success and failure.

We do promise that fidgeting can make a difference in your life. It can produce that extra weight loss that brings you to or near your goal when previously you had been falling short, even with dieting *and* exercise, no matter what you did. It can mean keeping your weight at a desired level instead of seeing it slowly pushing the digits or needle on your scale further along.

A PEEK INTO YOUR FUTURE

Trudy Fortunato swears by fidgeting. But just a few months ago she was ready to swear at everybody and everything in her path, so frustrated had she become over her efforts to lose weight. A flight attendant based in Chicago, Trudy had virtually forsaken her beloved fudge brownies for an artificial approximation of her treat that the local health food store carried. Aside from a few slips, she had followed the rest of her diet pretty faithfully.

Exercise was part of her job—or haven't you noticed flight attendants pushing those heavy refreshment carts uphill as you sit back in your seat and soar into the friendly skies? She also supplemented her work-time workout with jogging three times a week and hitting the exercise bike when her schedule permitted.

She wasn't doing too badly at her weekly weigh-in. Between losing a pound here and putting back a little there, she was slightly ahead of the game. But her goal of losing fifteen pounds always seemed to loom ahead of her like some insurmountable hurdle. The closer it got, the harder it looked. The difficulty Trudy was having in taking off—and keeping off—those last few pounds, which kept coming and going from her frame, was really getting her down. But after a while she made it over the top. She did it not by adding a major exercise to her schedule but by stepping up the frequency of scores of little things she already did throughout the day and adding a few new but simple twists. For example, when she arrived early for a flight or the aircraft was delayed, she sat down and jiggled her legs up and down, a slightly nervous gesture she had had for years, but now she was doing it on purpose.

During the flight, when Trudy wasn't picking up or pushing or holding something, she kept a rubber band doubled around her fingers, which she flexed against the resistance. When she was home, she took advantage of her tendency to wave her arms while she was talking on the phone. All it took was holding one of her son's baseballs in her free hand to turn a simple gesture into an exercise.

This is an example of what we mean by fidgeting as a factor in weight control. Through all these minor, really trivial, bits of physical activity, slipped in between everything else she was doing during the day, Trudy was burning 400 calories per day more than before she started. Not an enormous amount if that was the extent of her physical activity, to be sure, but a significant amount on top of everything else she did—enough to make the difference she was looking for.

Imagine a minor but unexpected financial windfall putting you ahead of the game or making up for some of your own deficit spending by helping you to pay off a few debts. Well, the calories you can burn from fidgeting can be that extra amount that brings you to your goal, or the safety net that saves you from yourself and the consequences of that birthday party where your self-control at the dessert table just melted like the icing on the cake.

Remember, you can fidget to burn calories no matter what the weather and can take advantage of the fidget factor even when you're home sick from work. You can fit fidgeting into the narrowest of time slots and you can do it even while you're busy doing something else—talking on the phone, for example, or vacuuming the house. There's no need to buy expensive equipment—in fact, you don't need anything you don't already have. Nor do you need a personal trainer or weekly classes. All you

YOU LIKE NUMBERS?

We've got some numbers—the amount of calories you can burn by just a little fidgeting. Each calorie expenditure is for ten minutes of that activity by a person weighing 130 pounds:

Sitting at your desk, crossing and uncrossing your legs: 20 calories

Standing on line, clasping your hands behind your back, then bringing your arms back to your sides: 15

Lying in bed watching TV, steadily changing your position: 14

Sitting at the kitchen table speaking on the phone, constantly rolling a rubber ball on the table with your free hand: 14

Now think about one of the more strenuous things you might do in the realm of formal exercise, such as riding a bike at ten miles an hour, also for ten minutes, that also add up to about 63 calories.

Suddenly those minuscule fidgeting routines begin to look a little more substantial, don't they? Imagine how many extra, bonus calories you could be burning if you were weaving similar activities into your entire day. A fidget here and a fidget there and suddenly you're getting someplace.

need is the desire to burn more calories than you already do and the commitment to look for and recognize the opportunities all around you to do so.

FIDGET, DON'T FUDGE IT

Just as you would like to mold your figure into pleasing proportions, so you will need to keep your sense of proportion when fitting fidgeting into your overall weight-control plan. There's a good reason why we call this book *The Fidget Factor*. It is not *The Fidget Solution, The Fidget Buster*, or *The Fidgeting-When-Nothing-Else-Has-Worked-and-You-Need-the-One-True-Answer-or-You'll-Die Book*.

STRIKE UP THE BAND

Fidgeting may not be magic, but waving a wand would be a good way to burn calories. If magic as a hobby is not your thing, another activity also involves waving something, but in this case to the beat of music: conducting. We hope you're not going to say that you've never waved your arms to conduct music coming from your stereo, especially when nobody was around. Everybody has probably done that at one time or another, maybe even without intending to when the music has really grabbed them. Well, there's no law that says you can't conduct on purpose.

So if music is your thing, find something around the house to serve as a baton. A ruler will do, maestro, but you can also buy a real, inexpensive baton from the local music store. "Conducting" your stereo is relaxing, it's fun, and you can really get into the music. Best of all, if you weigh 143 pounds and do it every day for just ten minutes, you will be burning 53 extra calories!

If fidgeting alone could solve all your problems, it would be magic. But the reason you are reading this book is almost certainly that all the weight-reduction methods you tried in the past promised too much and delivered too little or not at all. You don't create a new and better you by putting yourself into the realm of sorcery—you do it by getting real.

Later on in the book we will show you just how fidgeting makes sense only in the context of a healthy eating plan and exercise regimen. We hope that you will stick with us for the *whole* picture.

Now enough of preliminaries. You want to get closer and quicker to a better you. So as a fidgeter we know once said, "Let's shake a leg and get to it!"

CHAPTER 2

THE FIDGET FACTOR

DID AN ELEMENTARY SCHOOL TEACHER EVER TELL YOU or a classmate to "sit still"? In fact, you couldn't do that literally. The human nervous system doesn't permit total absence of motion. But we've seen some couch potatoes who can achieve a remarkable approximation of this placid state. Except for the slight tremor of a finger, the throb of a pulse—assuming they're still alive—or the twitch of an eyebrow, they have their gears in PARK and they have curbed their expenditure of energy to the max. All except when they have to push a button on the remote, of course.

Such a condition is nothing to brag about unless you are a mystic trying to put yourself into a trance. Movement is a natural state for all living creatures. Like breathing and eating, it plays an important role in the process by which we make use of our environment to sustain life.

If there's one essential nugget of new information we hope you take from this book, it's the value of *almost any kind of movement* in maintaining fitness and good health. It is no accident that the American Heart Association's fitness Web site can be found at this address: www.justmove. org. Note that they're not pushing weight lifting, working

11

A RESTFUL NIGHT'S SLEEP

Even when you sleep, you're on the move. You don't believe that? In the early days of television, a popular program called *You Asked for It* tracked down the answers to questions sent in by viewers. The subject matter ranged from historical curiosities to odd aspects of nature. In one of the most memorable episodes, a viewer asked if it was true that during a typical night's sleep people changed positions enough times to make it seem like they were doing nocturnal calisthenics. To answer him, the producers went to a prominent sleep laboratory, where they rigged up a camera to record a volunteer's night of "restful" sleep. The film, speeded up to encapsulate eight hours into a few minutes, was a revelation. The volunteer looked as if he was dancing to a swing band, so active was his sound sleep.

out to tighten your abs, stepping, jogging, or high-board diving. They're just emphasizing the importance of moving. Anything but lying on the couch in a TV-induced stupor.

Unfortunately, most people don't move most of the time. For too many of us, our days are filled with inactivity. In the workplace, sitting in one spot all day is a major problem. In the home, labor-saving appliances and entertainment systems that put the world at our fingertips are another obstacle to movement.

If this sounds a little abstract, why not create an activity profile of yourself? Keep a log of your day, recording how long you sit in one place and remain essentially motionless. Do it for at least one weekday and one Sunday, and then repeat both days in at least three separate weeks to get a reliable average.

You might surprise yourself, although we should warn you that the surprise may not be too pleasant. For a living, breathing adult person, you're likely to discover that you

AN INACTIVE POPULATION

According to the Centers for Disease Control, 25 to 35 percent of adults in this country engage in no physical activity outside work, and more than 60 percent don't come up to the minimum level that would be likely to keep a person healthy—thirty minutes of moderate activity, five days a week. People most at risk for being too inactive are women ages eighteen to forty-five who are married with children. Not surprisingly, they are least likely to be active in the winter months.

spend an awful lot of time resembling a bump on a log. If so, you are too typically American.

DO *WHAT?*

No matter how physically active you are now, we would like to move you into introducing some gentle yet calorie-burning activities into every nook and cranny of your busy life. Or to put it another way: *How would you like to put your body to work gradually consuming extra calories in the background, every day, while you get on with the rest of your life?*

Did you ever notice how frequently people who have nervous mannerisms such as folding and unfolding their arms, putting a hand to the back of their heads, touching their knees, and shifting in their seats tend to be thin? Not all the time but often enough to make it look like a pattern? In fact, there may be something more than chance behind it.

In January 1999, Drs. James Levine, Norman Eberhardt, and Michael D. Jensen, endocrinologists at the Mayo Clinic, published an article in *Science* describing a study they performed with sixteen people, twelve men and four women, who were observed over two months at the Mayo Clinic. These subjects had responded to an announcement that the clinic had posted asking for volunteers prepared to overeat for the sake of science.

The volunteers, who were largely sedentary but not obese, didn't have to work too hard. In fact, they were specifically told to minimize exercise, even though they had 1,000 calories a day added to their diet, a situation the subjects likened to experiencing Thanksgiving every day.

The experiment was carefully controlled. The research team monitored the subjects' physical activity—they wore pedometers to record how far they walked—and even scrutinized their garbage to make sure they ate everything they were supposed to, including dessert.

The food that contributed the 1,000 extra calories a day—40 percent carbohydrates, 40 percent fat, and 20 percent protein, the equivalent of eating two Big Macs a day—was meant to add pounds to their frames, and add it did. By the end of the two months, each of the subjects had gained anywhere from two to sixteen pounds. Now here's the crux of the matter: Why the disparity? What were those who gained less doing to ward off the effects of this caloric onslaught?

Jensen, Eberhardt, and Levine adjusted the results for differences in metabolism through a process called indirect calorimetry and also determined how much of the extra calories each individual had converted to fat to isolate the factor that was serving as some kind of mysterious fitness fairy godmother for some, while leaving the others to get nothing but fatter. The calories that had been burned that could not be accounted for by metabolism or conversion to fat had to have been consumed through some other process.

Here's what they found. On average, each subject did the following with that surplus of 1,000 calories a day:

39 percent ended up as body fat; 4 percent became body tissue other than fat; 14 percent was used in the process of digesting and storing the food; 8 percent was accounted for by basal metabolism—energy burned when you're doing nothing but lying down or sitting and breathing.

That left the researchers with about one-third of the calories unaccounted for. There was only one thing that could be consuming them: fidgeting. Some of the subjects fidgeted more than others—not on purpose, but rather because they did so characteristically. In effect, although told not to exercise, the volunteers who showed the least weight gain were burning off the calories in spite of themselves. *One man actually got rid of 700 of those 1,000 extra calories a day by fidgeting, an amount equivalent to what you might burn by jogging seven miles.*

Without intending to, the subjects who fidgeted were doing very moderate, minute exercises, engaging in almost constant movement so slight that most people would not label it "exercise." If you had asked these lucky people what they were "doing," they would probably have replied, "Nothing."

Of course, being scientists, Drs. Levine, Eberhardt, and Jensen weren't going to call this exactly nothing. What they called it was nonexercise activity thermogenesis, or NEAT.

People for whom NEAT is natural are apparently able to switch it on without thinking, to fidget more when they eat more to compensate for excess calories consumed. But if you are NEAT-impaired and overeat, your body converts the excess calories into fat unless you engage in an exercise program to burn off the surplus calories.

If NEAT promotes weight control, and therefore good health, why hasn't it become a natural part of every human being's activity profile—wouldn't it be a factor in evolution, helping members of the species to survive? There is no answer to that question, although, as noted in *Science News*, Elliot Danforth, professor emeritus, of the Department of Medicine at the University of Vermont has speculated that in the not-too-distant past, when famine was more prevalent as a cyclical occurrence in human affairs, not fidgeting and thus not "wasting" excess energy could have bolstered a baby's chances of survival.

While not speculating on the precise way that fidgeting might fit into an all-inclusive weight-control plan that included heavier exercise as well as low-level physical activities, such as those we discussed in the previous chapter, Jensen, Eberhardt, and Levine specified that such a routine seemed reasonable. In fact, they concluded their report in *Science* by suggesting "that efforts to enhance NEAT activation, perhaps through behavioral clues, may be a fruitful approach to the prevention of obesity."

WHAT'S IN IT FOR YOU

The Mayo Clinic's Dr. Michael D. Jensen would be the first to caution that fidgeting is not a panacea for the temptations of the table or a substitute for the exercise you haven't done but intend to do. You're sure to "burn a lot more calories with even a brief exercise program than you will by just fidgeting in your chair," he cautioned in a May 1999 article in *Vegetarian Times*. You still need to watch what you eat and engage in at least moderately vigorous activities such as walking.

CHEW THE FAT AWAY

In a December 1999 letter published in *The New England Journal of Medicine*, Dr. James Levine of the Mayo Clinic suggested that chewing gum may actually aid in the fight against fat.

Seven people with normal, stable weights were recruited for the clinic's experiment. The subjects sat in a dark, silent laboratory, and researchers measured the energy they expended at rest for thirty minutes, then the energy expended while chewing sugarless gum for twelve minutes, and finally the energy expended for twelve minutes after chewing. What the study showed was that gum chewing helped burn an extra eleven calories per hour. That may not sound like many calories, but consider this: If a person chewed sugarless gum constantly throughout the day (except at meals and while sleeping), he or she could conceivably lose eleven pounds a year. Talk about chewing the fat!

Nevertheless, according to Jensen, "every calorie that you burn by moving around counts. There's a range of extra calories that we can burn every day. If you increase that range a little bit, you're going to tend to stay leaner than if you just sit still and do nothing."

You may already know that moderate, low-level exercise activities such as walking or biking regularly, climbing stairs, doing yard work, and making repairs around the house are as much calorie burners as using a rowing machine, lifting free weights, and jogging. (We will have a good deal more to say about this later.) They're not as good for adding muscle nor are they nearly as effective as more strenuous activities for aerobic conditioning, but they are just as effective for keeping weight off, with the proviso that you manage to cobble together a combination of regular moderate exercise activities that burns the equivalent number of calories that would be consumed by the more strenuous activities of a formal workout.

What the Mayo Clinic study on fidgeting has done is to supply the last, and in some ways the most useful, link in the chain, tying together a broad spectrum of movement from heavy exercise to low-level exercise to fidgeting that could be consciously employed for weight control. The newest twist is that *all* movement short of an actual workout, especially moderate, low-level exercise combined with fidgeting, could prove to be a valuable and, what's more important, a *workable* way of burning calories that either supplements formal workouts or that substitutes for them when going to the gym or using exercise equipment at home is not feasible or is just too inconvenient.

But how does fidgeting fit into this scheme? How could you benefit from it? What if you are just not a fidgety kind of person? Hold relatively still for just a moment and we'll show you how you can fidget with the best of them.

FEELING FIDGETY?

First let's make our definitions clear. There is no exact dividing line between low-level exercise and fidgeting as purposeful, calculated movement. Nor does fidgeting as exercise have to be—nor should it be—confined to the conscious use of what we might otherwise regard as nervous mannerisms. For our purposes, fidgeting is simply movement that usually drops below the threshold of even low-level exercise and one's daily activities. Fidgeting is getting up and pacing while you're on the phone, stretching your arms over your head while gazing out the window (deep in thought, of course), and swinging your legs up and down under your desk while at work. Fidgeting can also begin to shade into exercise as desktop calisthenics, or involve enhancement of everyday movements by the application of resistance, such as wearing wrist weights around the house.

Fidgeting consists of movements that burn relatively few calories at a time, but that if done with any consistency throughout the day, add up to a significant contribution to your weight-control program over the course of the day and week, a weapon against fat you had all along but never realized you could activate.

"Activate?" As in *consciously* fidgeting? Doing this, er, involuntary thing on purpose? Certainly it sounds odd at first to think that you can learn to fidget, train yourself to fidget, want to fidget. If you've previously associated fidgeting simply with a person who can't sit still, you might naturally have a negative reaction. At best, it could sound silly and at worst, well, it could sound silly.

If you feel that way, give it another name: NEAT training, the Weight Mastery Through Movement Program, minimal-movement workouts. Does that sound better? The simple fact is that fidgeting burns calories and all calories are created equal. Why should you care where they come from? The calories you burn here are added to any you burn through more strenuous activities—or at least help substitute for those calories normally expended via sweat when circumstances prevent you from doing heavier exercise. Any way you look at it, they are calories that are gone, and good riddance!

THE PHILOSOPHY OF FIDGETING

Fidgeting is not only an activity, but a kind of physical outlook on life that says all things being equal, it's better to move, even if it's a little bit. For example, when you get to the airport, do you walk or opt for the people mover? If there's a wait for your flight, do you park yourself in one of those black-cushioned seats and watch CNN on the overhead screen, or do you walk—pace is more like it—around the immediate area of the terminal, checking out the shops, the newsstand, the arrival and departure information on the terminal screens? If it's the latter, you're burning three times the number of calories as the person who goes right for the seat. And, what the heck, once you get on the plane, you'll have all the sitting you can handle anyway, right?

When you end up standing on a line, do you just sort of droop and at most fold your arms in resignation, or do you shift your weight from foot to foot, hold the paper and read it, take out some knitting, stretch your arms behind you and then in front and then overhead? How about when you have to get to the next floor—do you take the stairs or the escalator or the elevator?

What do you do when you're on the phone? Do you just sit and talk? Or do you get up and pace, stabbing the air as you make a point, shrugging your shoulders in reaction to what the other person is saying, gesturing as you would if the person to whom you are speaking were in the room with you?

Yes, many people do these things as a matter of second nature. Such instinctive movement may not be you in the sense of ingrained responses to situations. But they're not complicated or weird. It's really just a kind of behavior that can be learned. You can *do* it. You don't have to do it all the time, but you can probably see the possibilities of learning it, just as you might learn to walk for thirty minutes a day, every day—and like it—even if you've never exercised before.

YOUR BASIC DAY

Here's how a typical day breaks down for an average man and woman:

Sleeping and resting: 8 hours

Sitting: 6

Standing: 6

Walking: 2

Activities a bit more active than walking: 2

About 75 percent of this day involves very low energy activities. Sitting and standing time, especially, is ripe for energy-enhancement so that it might be more productive in terms of calories burned. The results of such a boost could be impressive when you realize that the difference between an active and a sedentary person is as little as an extra hour a day of increased physical activity.

In the following pages, we're going to ask you to look at your daily routine with the aim of finding opportunities to add fidgeting to it. Please remember that these are just suggestions about what you might do and an orientation toward how to look at what you do each day so that you will eventually devise the kind of "fidgeting" that fits you best.

LOOK AROUND YOU

Okay, maybe you can learn to make use of fidgeting. Where do you start? The best place to begin is where you are. For most people, that means at home or at work. Look for the possibilities. If you are inclined to make lists, make a few to give you a sense of where you will be and what you are likely to be doing during a typical day. (See chapter 4 for a handy log you can use for this purpose.) Be particularly alert to the way that fidgeting activities can end up serving dual purposes, as you will quickly see from the ones we suggest.

What *do* you do every day? You bathe, for one thing. In the shower, you could grab one of those long back massagers and scrub yourself in rhythm. Alternate between pulling the massager back and forth and holding it still while you wiggle your body against it. When you soap yourself, do it vigorously—humming helps to get you in the mood. When you shampoo your hair, give yourself a good scalp massage. That will really wake you up and relax you at the same time, as well as burn extra calories and exercise your fingers.

Once you're out of the tub or shower stall, give it a quick cleaning. Yes, it could probably wait until Saturday, but there will be one less chore on the weekend if you break it up into small cleaning jobs during the week, and you will be exercising quite a few muscles while you're at it. Meanwhile, the tub or stall will stay clean all the time.

Surely you brush your teeth when you get up in the morning. We don't know anyone who finds that interesting. But what if you paced back and forth while you did it? When you get tired of doing that, stay in front of the sink but shift your weight from one foot to the other. If you're musically inclined, do it in rhythm. You could also be going over that idea you wanted to suggest later to your supervisor—moving leads to creative thinking. Or you could just rehash the last good move in that chess game the night before.

Then it's down to breakfast. What if you didn't resort to orange juice in the carton? Hand-squeezing oranges will not only provide you with a more nutritious drink— after all, much of what you want from that orange, aside from the taste, is in the pulp—but will also allow you to begin your day working off a few calories.

Do you see how the calorie expenditure is already beginning to slowly mount up? True, any one of these extra or embellished activities will lead you to use an amount of calories that will not get out of the lower double digits. But add them up—and you are just greeting the day at this point—and they will look like real numbers by bedtime. Promise!

While you're in the kitchen, consider all those labor-saving appliances, the side effects of which may be showing up as love handles and other unwanted protuberances. What if you did something really strange to combat that, something truly wild and primitive that would get your friends talking? Try washing your dishes by hand. You don't have to do it for every meal, just a few times a week makes a difference. Revolutionary! While you're at it, unless you're in a huge hurry, dry them as well.

At the stove or the sink, no matter what you're doing, rock back and forth (unless, of course, you are holding a pot of scalding hot liquid). Got a few spare minutes while something boils, broils, or bakes? Here's some genuine exercise to fill the time, although you will improvise the props from what's at hand. Grab a couple of cans of soup from the pantry and use them as dumb-bells, lifting them up and down, swinging them back and forth, even punching the air with them. Figure out how much time like this you might productively fill in the kitchen each week. Then multiply that by 50 or so and you'll get an idea of how many calories you could knock off in a year.

Don't confine your kitchen fidgeting to adding a twist to things you already do. Take fidgeting as an invitation to add new dishes to your repertoire that, coincidentally, might provide you with some calorie-burning opportunities. For example, do you like the smell of warm bread? Just about everyone does. If you've never had the pleasure of baking your own, now is a wonderful time to start. Kneading the dough is a real calorie cruncher, yet it's also soothing and many people swear by it. However, one caveat: Don't take this up if you think you might consume most of your bread yourself, because that would be ridiculously counterproductive. If you think that's a real danger, perhaps you could bake only when you're expecting company—in which case, maybe you need to invite friends over more often.

With so many home cooks and restaurants serving instant mashed potatoes these days, the real thing is at quite a premium. Nobody seems to want to do what it takes to reduce potatoes to the right consistency by hand anymore. Imagine how much your guests and family—and you, too—would appreciate that special taste if you took the trouble to mash them the old-fashioned way. If you need to be motivated, imagine, as well, the calories you will burn while doing it. In fact, that's a good thought to have to motivate yourself while you're mashing.

HOUSEWORK

How about turning your housework into a musical? Well, we're exaggerating a bit, but you could put your favorite CD on the stereo and

- Dance while you dust. It's about the only thing that could lift this mundane, humdrum chore out of anything more than the level of sheer necessity for survival.

- Swing and sway as you carry the wash from one place to another, even do a little stutter step. Gently swing the basket out in front of you and then pull it back to the beat. If it's not too big and heavy, lift it over your head a couple of times. Eventually you may end up doing this automatically, without having to think about it.

- Scrub the floors back and forth in time to the music. We won't promise that this chore will suddenly become fun, but it can at least begin to pay off with more calories burned from increased intensity as you rub. The same goes for the kitchen and bathroom sink.

TIME OUT

Did you ever stop to look at that word "recreation"? You're supposed to be re-creating something, as in reviving, refreshing, renewing. Lying on the couch motionless hardly fits the bill. If you absolutely must do that when you're watching TV or listening to music, then you're probably not getting enough sleep at night. Here are some better ways to re-create yourself during your leisure time:

- Sit up when you watch TV—it burns more calories than staying prone.

- Shift your position every few minutes while you watch. It's better for your back and all your joints. You don't have to turn into a fidgety fanatic: Just move a bit, turn, maybe stretch a little while you do it. Here's an easy way you can remember to shift: Do it every time there's a commercial break or a pause between selections on a CD.

- Get up and walk over to the TV when you change the channel. There's enough remoteness already in modern life without letting a remote control govern your existence. It's all those remote controls that may be helping your weight to go out of control in the first place.

- Find other things to do while you watch TV. Doing chores such as folding the laundry and peeling and cutting up vegetables for dinner burns calories and makes more efficient use of the time in your tightly scheduled day.

- Sit up or lean on your side when reading in bed, supporting yourself on an elbow: It uses up more energy than remaining flat on your back—anything does. Reading a book is also easier over time if you regularly shift its position.

- Have a pillow fight with your mate (put the book down first, please). You don't need an occasion (but be careful about doing this when you're angry).

- Give your mate a vigorous massage. Now there's an activity that produces multiple benefits all around, from burning calories to flexing joints to emotional contentment to raising the subject of sex. Among the many kinds of physical activities, sex is a rather nice way of burning calories—at least 80 or so. The exact amount depends—it's not what you do, but the way you do it. If we have to start enumerating the additional benefits to be gained from *that*, you're reading the wrong book.

OUT AND ABOUT

Fidgeting's place is not just in the home, although clearly you might want to be circumspect about a few things when you're in public. Wiggling and dancing by yourself, for example, are usually not good choices. Yet there are plenty of opportunities to stretch and flex and move without standing out in a crowd, and you can identify them if you just know where to look.

For example, you're in the doctor's or dentist's waiting room. Inquire as soon as you arrive as to how long the wait is likely to be. If it's substantial—and in the age of HMOs, that's becoming the rule—don't just hang around. Put your things in the closet and go out for a walk, even if it's just around the block. If you're lucky to catch the doc on a good day and the wait will be no worse than moderate, you can still go out in the hall and do a little stretching. People duck out for cigarettes all the time, so you can certainly do it for this more healthful reason.

While sitting and browsing through *People* or *Newsweek*, cross and uncross your legs. Hold the magazine folded with one hand, then open with two. Flex your neck and your arms. Every time you feel compelled to look up at the clock or at your watch—and you just know you will be doing that—take it as a signal for a "time" break. Get up and walk over to the window and stand for a while. Even if you have to fill out some forms, do it standing at the counter or window instead of sitting down.

Here are other opportunities to keep moving:

- Standing on a corner waiting for the light to turn green. Back exercises are especially helpful to offset the strain on your back that walking can sometimes cause. You can do one of them, the pelvic tilt, while "standing still." Just stand up straight and tuck and tilt in your abdomen a few times. Hold for a slow count of 5. Alternate that with squeezing your buttocks. Flex your shoulders to support your upper back and keep from getting a stiff neck: Holding your arms at midchest, move your elbows back behind you. Always keep breathing during these micromaneuvers.

- Standing on line. What do you usually do when you get trapped in place like that? You could be moving while keeping your place on line. Try some toe lifts, for example. Slowly stand up on tiptoe, then ease down. Mix this in with shifting your weight from one foot to the other, swinging your arms back and forth, rocking back and forth, and moving your head around in a small arc so that you feel a rolling motion in your neck. This almost-perpetual motion will not only keep your muscles and joints from getting stiff, burning calories in the process, but also make the time go faster.

- Meeting a friend for lunch or dinner at a restaurant. If the weather permits, wait outside, not inside at the bar or at a table. Right off the bat, you are probably achieving a kind of negative gain because you won't be tempted to have a drink or a snack or to start nibbling at the bread basket until your friend shows up. Once you're standing around outside, you can fidget in the way we described above for waiting at a corner for the light to change. If you get there really early, go window shopping, frequently doubling back to the restaurant to see if your friend has shown up early, too.

- Buying a book. The Internet and World Wide Web have made shopping for many things a breeze. The trouble is that when you use your computer to shop, you never get to feel so much as a breeze. Take books, for example. You probably don't have to go any further than Amazon.com to get what you want. But is the book itself all you want? When was the last time you were in a book store? Remember how much fun it was to browse? If you spent some time there, you probably had to bend and squat quite a bit when looking for something on a lower shelf. Today's huge national chains, such as Border's and Barnes and Noble, have such big stores that just wandering around in them begins to burn calories. Make it a point of doing at least some of your shopping for books with your feet rather than your fingers.

ON YOUR WAY TO WORK

Why wait until you get to the office to fidget? If you commute by car, start there. No matter what your route, you will surely have to wait for at least a few traffic lights, and if you live in a heavily populated suburb or city, there's also a good chance that you will encounter some bumper-to-bumper traffic at either end of the rush hour. So even if you're the one who's driving, there will be some time that you will spend just sitting—or fidgeting, the choice is yours.

Okay, the traffic is backed up for a mile near the new construction site and you've come to a dead stop, possibly for five minutes or more. What do you actually *do* now that the opportunity is here?

- Fold your hands on the back of your neck and then swing one elbow forward at a time. Vary the pace. If you're listening to music, keep time. Since you will be sitting for a while, a little flexing would therefore be good for your joints.

- Place your hands on the steering wheel and lift one elbow up at a time.

- Hold both hands in front of you and intertwine your fingers, turning them over so that your palms are pushing outward. Then stretch your palms forward over the steering wheel as far as you can, holding them out there for a few seconds before bringing them back.

- Shake hands with yourself; pull your hands apart but don't let go. When you feel a considerable amount of tension, hold it for a few seconds. And there you have it: traffic-jam isometrics.

- Swivel your hips, one side forward at a time, then the other. You can also rock from side to side, shrug your shoulders up and down, and swing one shoulder forward, then the other.

- Keep a small rubber ball in the glove compartment— just right to squeeze when the flow of traffic permits.

- Store a small plastic water bottle full of sand in the glove compartment to use as a weight, lift it up and down, one hand at a time.

- Drum your fingers on the steering wheel in time to music. Also try tapping your hands on your thighs as if you were playing bongo drums. Keep time as well by tapping your foot, assuming it's off the accelerator. You feel like singing? Sing. The odds are you will have the windows closed and nobody will hear you. If you're car-pooling, get the others to sing with you.

AT WORK

Make a resolution that unless you're in a hurry or working on a tight schedule, you will never get off the elevator at your floor. Always get off two or three floors before and use the stairs. But don't just walk up. You've just created another fidget time-slot. You're likely to be alone in the stairwell, so stop at each landing and raise your arms over your head, stretching just about as far as you can. Repeat the stretch five times. Then reach down with one arm as you raise the other. Switch arms.

Do you have papers delivered to your desk every morning—such as mail, memos, announcements, and sales figures? You could arrange to pick them up yourself. These days, most people understand if you tell them you're doing it to stretch your legs and get a little exercise.

For most people, their office or cubicle constitutes their main work environment. But just because you sit for most of the day, it doesn't mean you have to be sedentary. All of the kinds of fidgeting we've introduced for other places are relevant here. For instance, do a mixture of the following throughout the day whenever the pace of work permits: Shrug your shoulders, then roll them; pull your abdomen in and then let it out; do the pelvic tilt; cross and uncross your arms; do the same with your legs; put your hands on your hips and swing one elbow forward while the other goes back and then reverse them; clasp your hands behind your head and twist from the hips one way and then the other. You're probably getting the picture. Also remember to change your position frequently when sitting, for the sake of your back as well as to burn a few more calories through the day.

Many people have jobs that allow them to listen to background music, perhaps through earphones, during part of the day. If you're one of those fortunate ones, keep an empty stapler on your desk and whenever one hand is free, use it to push on the stapler in time to the music.

Think about how much time you spend on the phone each workday. You don't need more than one hand to hold the receiver, giving you a golden opportunity to do something useful with the other that will at least expend a few calories. Without missing a beat, you could be "talking" with your free hand—perhaps pacing back and forth while you hand-talk. If it appeals to you, you could keep one of those small hand-dexterity games on your desk to pass time on the phone actively, the kind of game where you have to roll a ball into one hole while avoiding another. Then there's your computer mouse: Put that plastic rodent to work, swirling it around in circles while you talk.

When was the last time you played with a yo-yo? You need only one hand. (But do put it away when you have visitors, who may not appreciate your serious purpose.) Here are a few more ideas:

- Keep a heavy paperweight on your desk and lift it up and down while you speak on the phone.

- Wave your free arm in the air while you make your points in the conversation, switching arms every minute or so. You may find that doing this helps you concentrate and come across more strongly than when you just sit there and talk.

- With your free hand, reach as far above your head as you can, hold it there for a few seconds, and then bring it as far down as you can.

- Keep a rubber ball either on your desk or in a drawer. Place it on top of the desk when the phone rings or when you make a call and put the palm of your free hand on the ball. Now roll it around in circles and back and forth for the length of the conversation.

- Always keep a couple of rubber bands nearby and while on the phone, place them over the fingers of your free hand so that they create a considerable resistance to spreading your fingers. Now slowly stretch your fingers and hold them out against the pressure of the rubber bands for a few seconds. Relax your fingers for a few seconds and then do it again. If you get tired of doing that, twirl a pencil.

No matter what you're doing on top of your desk, your feet can always be busy expending calories below it. Get a slightly larger ball than you use on top of the desk—a soccer ball or volleyball would be just right—and put it on the floor underneath. Regularly, throughout the day, keep one foot on it and roll the ball around. Switch feet frequently. You could also strengthen your thighs by occasionally putting the ball between your legs and squeezing it.

You could also lift your feet up and down as if you were walking; lift one foot off the floor and swing it around, then do the same with the other foot; and keep a foot pedal under your desk and pump it.

The odds are that your chair is on rollers. If so, put them to good use: Use your feet and legs to roll the chair back and forth and from side to side frequently during the day. Don't try to push it very far—just enough so that you feel your leg muscles doing a little work. You wouldn't do this while typing, naturally, but you would be surprised at how large a percentage of the day your work would permit this activity. After a while, you may find that the rolling rhythm also serves to relax you.

If you're ambitious, put on ankle weights whenever you're going to be at your desk for some time. Then do all these routines with extra poundage on your legs, possibly as much as doubling the calories you were burning before.

When you have to spend most of the day at your desk, you will have to take breaks from the computer anyway about every forty-five minutes, so why not indulge in a little desk yoga to get in some stretching? Believe it or not, there is such a thing as keyboard yoga and you can find the easy diagrams that show you how to do it with just a quick search of the Internet.

Unless you are high up in your organization, you may have to make your own copies and get printouts from a network printer yourself. If you do, you are among the lucky ones, because it's another occasion to get up and take a walk down the hall. Others would do well to emulate you, stretching their legs and letting the administrative assistants do more important things (such as actually run the organization, which many of them do).

Similarly, you could have lunch sent in, especially if you are up to your neck in work and feel you have time only to grab a bite at your desk. But literally working nonstop tends to be counterproductive. Eventually fatigue sets in and you do less than you could have if you had only taken mini-exercise breaks. A good compromise on lunch would be to go out and get it yourself but then bring it back and eat at your desk. That would give you a chance to take a walk, use the stairs, and maybe get some fresh air. Then you could come back refreshed and ready to plow right back into it.

Finally, there's E-mail. It's truly wonderful for communicating with colleagues in faraway places or at least when they're across town, but do you really need to use it when your correspondent is down at the other end of the hall or only a few floors away? E-mail is time-consuming to read and answer and often you could be putting that time to better use. Face-to-face meetings, whenever they are relevant, are more productive, lead to fewer misunderstandings, and have the added attraction of serendipity: New ideas emerge unexpectedly even when you hadn't intended to brainstorm. Better yet, you and your colleague might profit by taking a walk together.

LIGHTING A FIRE UNDER YOURSELF

We spent some time on motivation when we discussed heavier exercise because we know that it's not easy to keep to such regimens. Just because fidgeting and associated low-level exercises are often minute in intensity doesn't mean that you won't need to motivate yourself to do them. If anything, you may need to work harder at keeping up fidgeting than you do for activities such as weight lifting and jogging. Since the fidget factor, to be effective, depends upon an accumulation of small measures, many of them fitting into the cracks of a busy schedule, anything that begins to erode the small details could end up destroying the big picture. Pass up a few of the things you've been doing and pretty soon you could let the whole thing slide.

If fidgeting doesn't come naturally to you, you will have to constantly be reminded of your intention to do it, especially in the beginning. When you do much of your fidgeting in one particular place, you could set up reminders for yourself. Post-it notes and the like are useful for this purpose. Put a Post-it note to yourself about fidgeting on your car's dashboard. If you fidget at the computer—at work or at home—put the note on the side of the screen.

If you're not intimidated by installing new software, screen savers are available, sometimes as "freeware," that will allow you to enter your own message, which will be flashed on the screen, reminding you to fidget. You could link it to one of the sounds your computer can make, or even download something more appropriate from the Web. With all the multimedia elements creeping into the use of the Web, perhaps you can find a file that has an appropriate tune, such as the old rock 'n' roll songs "All Shook Up" and "Shake, Rattle and Roll."

At other times, you might want to use inanimate objects as mnemonic devices. For example, if when cooking you have one pot that you use more than others, associate it with all the fidgeting routines you do around the kitchen. Touching or even just seeing that pot becomes your cue to fidget. Likewise you could put something in your pants pocket—a token, an old coin, a key chain, anything that you will immediately recognize when you put your hand in your pocket—that can remind you to fidget when you're out for a walk.

THE POSSIBILITIES ARE ENDLESS

One of the great things about fidgeting is that it's so malleable. We've been making some suggestions just to give you an idea of what's involved and perhaps get you started. But by all means, make fidgeting your own. Customize it to your personality and interests, so you can create fidgeting moves that go with your daily activities, hobbies, and schedule. The table in chapter 3, which includes hundreds of things to do along with calorie expenditures by body weight, will help you plan your fidgeting.

Once you get used to looking for fidgeting opportunities, you will probably see them everywhere, even when you're lying in a hammock or stretched out on a chaise lounge. Eventually it could even color the way you feel about yourself. Getting going here could motivate you to end the inertia in other areas of your life. Before you know it, you could really feel you're on the move.

CHAPTER 3

CALORIE EXPENDITURE CHART

HOW TO USE THE CALORIE EXPENDITURE CHART

The following chart details the number of calories burned in household, occupational, sports, and physical fitness activities. While the list is by no means exhaustive, we've tried to include every common—and not-so-common—motion you might employ.

Determining the number of calories you can burn is easy. First, choose an activity from the chart. To the right of each activity is the number of calories burned per minute. Second, locate the body weight closest to your own. We've listed both kilograms and pounds. Third, multiply the number of calories burned per minute by the time spent performing that motion. For example, a 150-pound person will burn 108 calories playing miniature gold for a half hour (3.6 calories per minute multiplied by 30 minutes equals 108 calories burned).

If your exact weight is not on the chart, there's a simple equation to determine the calories burned per minute for your weight. Find the weight closest to yours on the chart and locate the number of calories burned per minute for that weight. For example, if you weigh 300 pounds and are trying to determine the number of calories burned during sleep, you would locate "Sleeping" on the chart and look up the rate for 262 pounds. That figure is 2.1 calories burned per minute. Multiply your weight (300) by the number of calories burned per minute (2.1) and divide by the weight closest to yours on the chart (262). In this instance, a 300-pound person burns 2.4 calories per minute while sleeping.

Calories Expended by Body Weight

Your Body Weight

Activity	kg lb	50 110	53 117	56 123	59 130	62 137	65 143	68 150	71 157	74 163
Accordion Playing		1.6	1.7	1.8	1.9	2.0	2.0	2.1	2.2	2.3
Aerobics—Dance										
General		5.3	5.6	5.9	6.2	6.5	6.8	7.1	7.5	7.8
High impact (class or using videotape)		7.8	8.3	8.8	9.3	9.7	10.2	10.7	11.1	11.6
High intensity–high impact (5 min. warmup, 20 min. routine; high impact requires both feet leave floor)		9.2	9.8	10.4	10.9	11.5	12.0	12.6	13.1	13.7
High intensity–low impact (5 min. warmup, 20 min. routine)		7.4	7.8	8.2	8.7	9.1	9.6	10.0	10.4	10.9
Low impact (116–148 beats/min.), wearing 1 lb hand weights, three 5 min. bouts		5.8	6.1	6.5	6.8	7.2	7.5	7.9	8.2	8.5
Low impact (136–148 beats/min.)		9.9	10.5	11.1	11.7	12.2	12.8	13.4	14.0	14.6
Low impact (class or using videotape)		6.3	6.7	7.0	7.4	7.8	8.2	8.5	8.9	9.3
Low impact, 9 min. bout		8.7	9.2	9.7	10.2	10.8	11.3	11.8	12.3	12.8
Low impact, wearing 1 lb hand weights, 9-min. bout		9.4	9.9	10.5	11.0	11.6	12.2	12.7	13.3	13.8
Low intensity–high impact (5 min. warmup, 20 min. routine)		8.0	8.5	9.0	9.4	9.9	10.4	10.9	11.4	11.8
Low intensity–low impact (5 min. warmup, 20 min. routine)		4.5	4.8	5.0	5.3	5.6	5.8	6.1	6.4	6.7
Teaching aerobic exercise (or fitness-type classes)		5.3	5.6	5.9	6.2	6.5	6.8	7.1	7.5	7.8
Water aerobics		3.5	3.7	3.9	4.1	4.3	4.6	4.8	5.0	5.2
Aerobics—Step (see also Bench Stepping)										
10 in. bench		7.0	7.4	7.8	8.2	8.6	9.1	9.5	9.9	10.3
JazzerStep; 6–8 in. bench (120 beats/min.)		7.7	8.1	8.6	9.0	9.5	10.0	10.4	10.9	11.3
Aqua-Running										
Wearing Aqua Jogger flotation belt, 48 strides/min., maximum effort		7.3	7.7	8.2	8.6	9.0	9.5	9.9	10.4	10.8

Calories Expended by Body Weight

Your Body Weight

77 170	80 176	83 183	86 190	89 196	92 203	95 209	98 216	101 223	104 229	107 236	110 243	113 249	116 256	119 262
2.4	2.5	2.6	2.7	2.8	2.9	3.0	3.1	3.2	3.3	3.4	3.5	3.6	3.7	3.7
8.1	8.4	8.7	9.0	9.3	9.7	10.0	10.3	10.6	10.9	11.2	11.6	11.9	12.2	12.5
12.1	12.6	13.0	13.5	14.0	14.4	14.9	15.4	15.9	16.3	16.8	17.3	17.7	18.2	18.7
14.2	14.8	15.4	15.9	16.5	17.0	17.6	18.1	18.7	19.2	19.8	20.3	20.9	21.5	22.0
11.3	11.8	12.2	12.6	13.1	13.5	14.0	14.4	14.8	15.3	15.7	16.2	16.6	17.1	17.5
8.9	9.2	9.6	9.9	10.3	10.6	11.0	11.3	11.7	12.0	12.4	12.7	13.1	13.4	13.7
15.2	15.8	16.4	17.0	17.6	18.2	18.8	19.4	20.0	20.5	21.1	21.7	22.3	22.9	23.5
9.7	10.0	10.4	10.8	11.2	11.5	11.9	12.3	12.7	13.0	13.4	13.8	14.2	14.6	14.9
13.4	13.9	14.4	14.9	15.5	16.0	16.5	17.0	17.5	18.1	18.6	19.1	19.6	20.1	20.7
14.4	15.0	15.5	16.1	16.6	17.2	17.8	18.3	18.9	19.5	20.0	20.6	21.1	21.7	22.3
12.3	12.8	13.3	13.8	14.2	14.7	15.2	15.7	16.2	16.6	17.1	17.6	18.1	18.6	19.0
6.9	7.2	7.5	7.7	8.0	8.3	8.5	8.8	9.1	9.4	9.6	9.9	10.2	10.4	10.7
8.1	8.4	8.7	9.0	9.3	9.7	10.0	10.3	10.6	10.9	11.2	11.6	11.9	12.2	12.5
5.4	5.6	5.8	6.0	6.2	6.4	6.7	6.9	7.1	7.3	7.5	7.7	7.9	8.1	8.3
10.7	11.2	11.6	12.0	12.4	12.8	13.3	13.7	14.1	14.5	14.9	15.3	15.8	16.2	16.6
11.8	12.3	12.7	13.2	13.6	14.1	14.6	15.0	15.5	15.9	16.4	16.9	17.3	17.8	18.2
11.2	11.7	12.1	12.5	13.0	13.4	13.8	14.3	14.7	15.2	15.6	16.0	16.5	16.9	17.3

Calories Expended by Body Weight

Your Body Weight

Activity	kg lb	50 110	53 117	56 123	59 130	62 137	65 143	68 150	71 157	74 163
Archery										
Hunting (walking)		3.7	3.9	4.1	4.3	4.6	4.8	5.0	5.2	5.4
Nonhunting, recreational		3.1	3.2	3.4	3.6	3.8	4.0	4.2	4.3	4.5
Arm Cranking										
Electromechanical ergometer, 60 rpm, maximum effort		12.3	13.1	13.8	14.6	15.3	16.0	16.8	17.5	18.3
Around the House: Bathroom										
Applying shampoo in rhythm		1.9	2.0	2.1	2.2	2.4	2.5	2.6	2.7	2.8
Brushing teeth: shifting weight foot to foot; pacing		2.3	2.4	2.6	2.7	2.9	3.0	3.1	3.3	3.4
Punching shower curtain		4.5	4.8	5.0	5.3	5.6	5.9	6.1	6.4	6.7
Scrubbing tub or shower stall		2.5	2.7	2.8	3.0	3.1	3.3	3.4	3.6	3.7
Shaking off moisture after bath or shower		2.2	2.3	2.5	2.6	2.7	2.9	3.0	3.1	3.3
Using back massager in rhythm		2.0	2.1	2.2	2.4	2.5	2.6	2.7	2.8	3.0
Vigorous soaping and rinsing		3.1	3.3	3.5	3.7	3.8	4.0	4.2	4.4	4.6
Around the House: Bedroom										
Changing position of book		0.9	1.0	1.0	1.1	1.1	1.2	1.2	1.3	1.3
Giving massage		1.7	1.8	1.9	2.0	2.1	2.2	2.3	2.4	2.5
Leaning on elbow		1.1	1.2	1.2	1.3	1.4	1.4	1.5	1.6	1.6
Lying on back, making pedaling motion with feet		1.9	2.0	2.1	2.2	2.4	2.5	2.6	2.7	2.8
Pillow fight		3.5	3.7	3.9	4.1	4.3	4.6	4.8	5.0	5.2
Shifting weight of book from hand to hand		0.9	1.0	1.0	1.1	1.1	1.2	1.2	1.3	1.3
Sitting up reading in bed		1.0	1.1	1.1	1.2	1.2	1.3	1.4	1.4	1.5
Standing up reading		1.6	1.7	1.8	1.9	2.0	2.1	2.2	2.3	2.4
Around the House: Housework										
Cleaning kitchen or bathroom sinks		4.8	5.1	5.4	5.7	6.0	6.2	6.5	6.8	7.1
Dancing while dusting		1.6	1.7	1.8	1.9	2.0	2.1	2.2	2.3	2.4
Dancing with a broom or vacuum cleaner		2.0	2.1	2.2	2.4	2.5	2.6	2.7	2.8	3.0
Doing squats		3.0	3.2	3.4	3.5	3.7	3.9	4.1	4.3	4.4

Calories Expended by Body Weight

Your Body Weight

77	80	83	86	89	92	95	98	101	104	107	110	113	116	119
170	176	183	190	196	203	209	216	223	229	236	243	249	256	262
5.7	5.9	6.1	6.3	6.5	6.8	7.0	7.2	7.4	7.6	7.9	8.1	8.3	8.5	8.7
4.7	4.9	5.1	5.3	5.5	5.6	5.8	6.0	6.2	6.4	6.6	6.7	6.9	7.1	7.3
19.0	19.7	20.5	21.2	22.0	22.7	23.4	24.2	24.9	25.7	26.4	27.1	27.9	28.6	29.4
2.9	3.0	3.2	3.3	3.4	3.5	3.6	3.7	3.8	4.0	4.1	4.2	4.3	4.4	4.5
3.5	3.7	3.8	4.0	4.1	4.2	4.4	4.5	4.6	4.8	4.9	5.1	5.2	5.3	5.5
6.9	7.2	7.5	7.7	8.0	8.3	8.6	8.8	9.1	9.4	9.6	9.9	10.2	10.4	10.7
3.9	4.0	4.2	4.3	4.5	4.6	4.8	4.9	5.1	5.2	5.4	5.5	5.7	5.8	6.0
3.4	3.5	3.7	3.8	3.9	4.0	4.2	4.3	4.4	4.6	4.7	4.8	5.0	5.1	5.2
3.1	3.2	3.3	3.4	3.6	3.7	3.8	3.9	4.0	4.2	4.3	4.4	4.5	4.6	4.8
4.8	5.0	5.1	5.3	5.5	5.7	5.9	6.1	6.3	6.4	6.6	6.8	7.0	7.2	7.4
1.4	1.4	1.5	1.5	1.6	1.7	1.7	1.8	1.8	1.9	1.9	2.0	2.0	2.1	2.1
2.6	2.7	2.8	2.9	3.0	3.1	3.2	3.3	3.4	3.5	3.6	3.7	3.8	3.9	4.0
1.7	1.8	1.8	1.9	2.0	2.0	2.1	2.2	2.2	2.3	2.4	2.4	2.5	2.6	2.6
2.9	3.0	3.2	3.3	3.4	3.5	3.6	3.7	3.8	4.0	4.1	4.2	4.3	4.4	4.5
5.4	5.6	5.8	6.0	6.2	6.4	6.7	6.9	7.1	7.3	7.5	7.7	7.9	8.1	8.3
1.4	1.4	1.5	1.5	1.6	1.7	1.7	1.8	1.8	1.9	1.9	2.0	2.0	2.1	2.1
1.5	1.6	1.7	1.7	1.8	1.8	1.9	2.0	2.0	2.1	2.1	2.2	2.3	2.3	2.4
2.5	2.6	2.7	2.8	2.8	2.9	3.0	3.1	3.2	3.3	3.4	3.5	3.6	3.7	3.8
7.4	7.7	8.0	8.3	8.5	8.8	9.1	9.4	9.7	10.0	10.3	10.6	10.8	11.1	11.4
2.5	2.6	2.7	2.8	2.8	2.9	3.0	3.1	3.2	3.3	3.4	3.5	3.6	3.7	3.8
3.1	3.2	3.3	3.4	3.6	3.7	3.8	3.9	4.0	4.2	4.3	4.4	4.5	4.6	4.8
4.6	4.8	5.0	5.2	5.3	5.5	5.7	5.9	6.1	6.2	6.4	6.6	6.8	7.0	7.1

Calories Expended by Body Weight

		Your Body Weight							
Activity	**kg 50** **lb 110**	**53** **117**	**56** **123**	**59** **130**	**62** **137**	**65** **143**	**68** **150**	**71** **157**	**74** **163**
Around the House: Housework (cont.)									
Swaying and doing a stutter step while carrying wash	1.7	1.8	1.9	2.0	2.1	2.2	2.3	2.4	2.5
Washing kitchen or bathroom floors	4.8	5.1	5.4	5.7	6.0	6.2	6.5	6.8	7.1
Around the House: Kitchen									
Baking bread and kneading dough	1.8	1.9	2.0	2.1	2.2	2.3	2.4	2.6	2.7
Chopping raw vegetables	1.7	1.8	1.9	2.0	2.1	2.2	2.3	2.4	2.5
Clearing table	2.0	2.1	2.2	2.4	2.5	2.6	2.7	2.8	3.0
Cooking standing up	2.1	2.2	2.4	2.5	2.6	2.7	2.9	3.0	3.1
Doing arm lifts using soup cans as weights	2.4	2.5	2.7	2.8	3.0	3.1	3.3	3.4	3.6
Drying the dishes	2.2	2.3	2.5	2.6	2.7	2.9	3.0	3.1	3.3
Making mashed potatoes by hand	1.5	1.6	1.7	1.8	1.9	2.0	2.0	2.1	2.2
Rocking back and forth	1.4	1.5	1.6	1.7	1.7	1.8	1.9	2.0	2.1
Washing dishes by hand	2.3	2.4	2.6	2.7	2.9	3.0	3.1	3.3	3.4
Around the House: Miscellaneous									
Dancing by yourself	4.1	4.3	4.6	4.8	5.1	5.3	5.6	5.8	6.1
Around the House: Watching TV									
Changing posture	1.2	1.3	1.3	1.4	1.5	1.6	1.6	1.7	1.8
Folding laundry	1.4	1.5	1.6	1.7	1.7	1.8	1.9	2.0	2.1
Holding 2–5 lb weight in each hand, doing arm curls rhythmically	3.0	3.2	3.4	3.5	3.7	3.9	4.1	4.3	4.4
Isometric exercises (straining or pushing against immovable object)	3.2	3.4	3.6	3.8	4.0	4.2	4.4	4.5	4.7
Sitting, tapping feet	1.6	1.7	1.8	1.9	2.0	2.1	2.2	2.3	2.4
Stretching slowly	2.2	2.3	2.5	2.6	2.7	2.9	3.0	3.1	3.3
Walking to TV to change channel, adjust volume	1.8	1.9	2.0	2.1	2.2	2.3	2.4	2.6	2.7
Around the House: You and the Kids									
Being soccer "goalie"	1.8	1.9	2.0	2.1	2.2	2.3	2.4	2.6	2.7
Carrying and setting up sports equipment	2.2	2.3	2.5	2.6	2.7	2.9	3.0	3.1	3.3
Crawling on floor with baby	1.8	1.9	2.0	2.1	2.2	2.3	2.4	2.6	2.7

Calories Expended by Body Weight

						Your Body Weight								
77 **170**	**80** **176**	**83** **183**	**86** **190**	**89** **196**	**92** **203**	**95** **209**	**98** **216**	**101** **223**	**104** **229**	**107** **236**	**110** **243**	**113** **249**	**116** **256**	**119** **262**
2.6	2.7	2.8	2.9	3.0	3.1	3.2	3.3	3.4	3.5	3.6	3.7	3.8	3.9	4.0
7.4	7.7	8.0	8.3	8.5	8.8	9.1	9.4	9.7	10.0	10.3	10.6	10.8	11.1	11.4
2.8	2.9	3.0	3.1	3.2	3.3	3.4	3.5	3.6	3.7	3.9	4.0	4.1	4.2	4.3
2.6	2.7	2.8	2.9	3.0	3.1	3.2	3.3	3.4	3.5	3.6	3.7	3.8	3.9	4.0
3.1	3.2	3.3	3.4	3.6	3.7	3.8	3.9	4.0	4.2	4.3	4.4	4.5	4.6	4.8
3.2	3.4	3.5	3.6	3.7	3.9	4.0	4.1	4.2	4.4	4.5	4.6	4.7	4.9	5.0
3.7	3.8	4.0	4.1	4.3	4.4	4.6	4.7	4.8	5.0	5.1	5.3	5.4	5.6	5.7
3.4	3.5	3.7	3.8	3.9	4.0	4.2	4.3	4.4	4.6	4.7	4.8	5.0	5.1	5.2
2.3	2.4	2.5	2.6	2.7	2.8	2.9	2.9	3.0	3.1	3.2	3.3	3.4	3.5	3.6
2.2	2.2	2.3	2.4	2.5	2.6	2.7	2.7	2.8	2.9	3.0	3.1	3.2	3.2	3.3
3.5	3.7	3.8	4.0	4.1	4.2	4.4	4.5	4.6	4.8	4.9	5.1	5.2	5.3	5.5
6.3	6.6	6.8	7.1	7.3	7.5	7.8	8.0	8.3	8.5	8.8	9.0	9.3	9.5	9.8
1.8	1.9	2.0	2.1	2.1	2.2	2.3	2.4	2.4	2.5	2.6	2.6	2.7	2.8	2.9
2.2	2.2	2.3	2.4	2.5	2.6	2.7	2.7	2.8	2.9	3.0	3.1	3.2	3.2	3.3
4.6	4.8	5.0	5.2	5.3	5.5	5.7	5.9	6.1	6.2	6.4	6.6	6.8	7.0	7.1
4.9	5.1	5.3	5.5	5.7	5.9	6.1	6.3	6.5	6.7	6.8	7.0	7.2	7.4	7.6
2.5	2.6	2.7	2.8	2.8	2.9	3.0	3.1	3.2	3.3	3.4	3.5	3.6	3.7	3.8
3.4	3.5	3.7	3.8	3.9	4.0	4.2	4.3	4.4	4.6	4.7	4.8	5.0	5.1	5.2
2.8	2.9	3.0	3.1	3.2	3.3	3.4	3.5	3.6	3.7	3.9	4.0	4.1	4.2	4.3
2.8	2.9	3.0	3.1	3.2	3.3	3.4	3.5	3.6	3.7	3.9	4.0	4.1	4.2	4.3
3.4	3.5	3.7	3.8	3.9	4.0	4.2	4.3	4.4	4.6	4.7	4.8	5.0	5.1	5.2
2.8	2.9	3.0	3.1	3.2	3.3	3.4	3.5	3.6	3.7	3.9	4.0	4.1	4.2	4.3

Calories Expended by Body Weight

					Your Body Weight				
Activity	**kg 50** **lb 110**	**53** **117**	**56** **123**	**59** **130**	**62** **137**	**65** **143**	**68** **150**	**71** **157**	**74** **163**
Around the House: You and the Kids (cont.)									
Hitting fly balls	2.4	2.5	2.7	2.8	3.0	3.1	3.3	3.4	3.6
Passing basketball	2.1	2.2	2.4	2.5	2.6	2.7	2.9	3.0	3.1
Picking up child and twirling	2.8	3.0	3.1	3.3	3.5	3.6	3.8	4.0	4.1
Playing catch tag	2.2	2.3	2.5	2.6	2.7	2.9	3.0	3.1	3.3
Pushing stroller (brisk walk)	3.2	3.4	3.6	3.8	4.0	4.2	4.4	4.5	4.7
Pushing stroller (slow walk)	2.7	2.9	3.0	3.2	3.3	3.5	3.7	3.8	4.0
Retrieving tennis balls	2.5	2.7	2.8	3.0	3.1	3.3	3.4	3.6	3.7
Running back and forth through sprinkler	2.3	2.4	2.6	2.7	2.9	3.0	3.1	3.3	3.4
Tossing football	2.4	2.5	2.7	2.8	3.0	3.1	3.3	3.4	3.6
Automobile Body Work	3.9	4.2	4.4	4.6	4.9	5.1	5.4	5.6	5.8
Automobile Repair	2.6	2.8	2.9	3.1	3.3	3.4	3.6	3.7	3.9
Backpacking (General)	6.2	6.6	7.0	7.4	7.7	8.1	8.5	8.8	9.2
Badminton									
Competition	6.1	6.5	6.9	7.2	7.6	8.0	8.3	8.7	9.1
Social singles and doubles	3.9	4.2	4.4	4.6	4.9	5.1	5.4	5.6	5.8
Baking (General)	3.5	3.7	3.9	4.1	4.3	4.6	4.8	5.0	5.2
Ballet—Classical									
Barre (20 min.), women	4.6	4.9	5.1	5.4	5.7	5.9	6.2	6.5	6.8
Barre (20 min.), men	4.6	4.9	5.1	5.4	5.7	6.0	6.2	6.5	6.8
Barre, high intensity (aerial jumps, midair turns, traveling steps (4 min.), women	5.9	6.2	6.6	6.9	7.3	7.6	8.0	8.3	8.7
Barre, high intensity (aerial jumps, midair turns, traveling steps (4 min.), men	6.6	7.0	7.4	7.8	8.2	8.6	8.9	9.3	9.7
Center-floor exercises, moderate intensity (6 min.), women	5.5	5.8	6.1	6.5	6.8	7.1	7.5	7.8	8.1
Ballroom Dancing									
Fast (disco, folk, square)	5.3	5.6	5.9	6.2	6.5	6.8	7.1	7.5	7.8
Slow (waltz, fox-trot, slow dancing)	3.1	3.2	3.4	3.6	3.8	4.0	4.2	4.3	4.5

Calories Expended by Body Weight

Your Body Weight

77 170	80 176	83 183	86 190	89 196	92 203	95 209	98 216	101 223	104 229	107 236	110 243	113 249	116 256	119 262
3.7	3.8	4.0	4.1	4.3	4.4	4.6	4.7	4.8	5.0	5.1	5.3	5.4	5.6	5.7
3.2	3.4	3.5	3.6	3.7	3.9	4.0	4.1	4.2	4.4	4.5	4.6	4.7	4.9	5.0
4.3	4.5	4.6	4.8	5.0	5.2	5.3	5.5	5.7	5.8	6.0	6.2	6.3	6.5	6.7
3.4	3.5	3.7	3.8	3.9	4.0	4.2	4.3	4.4	4.6	4.7	4.8	5.0	5.1	5.2
4.9	5.1	5.3	5.5	5.7	5.9	6.1	6.3	6.5	6.7	6.8	7.0	7.2	7.4	7.6
4.2	4.3	4.5	4.6	4.8	5.0	5.1	5.3	5.5	5.6	5.8	5.9	6.1	6.3	6.4
3.9	4.0	4.2	4.3	4.5	4.6	4.8	4.9	5.1	5.2	5.4	5.5	5.7	5.8	6.0
3.5	3.7	3.8	4.0	4.1	4.2	4.4	4.5	4.6	4.8	4.9	5.1	5.2	5.3	5.5
3.7	3.8	4.0	4.1	4.3	4.4	4.6	4.7	4.8	5.0	5.1	5.3	5.4	5.6	5.7
6.1	6.3	6.5	6.8	7.0	7.2	7.5	7.7	8.0	8.2	8.4	8.7	8.9	9.1	9.4
4.0	4.2	4.4	4.5	4.7	4.8	5.0	5.1	5.3	5.5	5.6	5.8	5.9	6.1	6.2
9.6	10.0	10.3	10.7	11.1	11.5	11.8	12.2	12.6	13.0	13.3	13.7	14.1	14.5	14.8
9.4	9.8	10.2	10.5	10.9	11.3	11.6	12.0	12.4	12.7	13.1	13.5	13.8	14.2	14.6
6.1	6.3	6.5	6.8	7.0	7.2	7.5	7.7	8.0	8.2	8.4	8.7	8.9	9.1	9.4
5.4	5.6	5.8	6.0	6.2	6.4	6.7	6.9	7.1	7.3	7.5	7.7	7.9	8.1	8.3
7.0	7.3	7.6	7.9	8.1	8.4	8.7	9.0	9.2	9.5	9.8	10.1	10.3	10.6	10.9
7.1	7.4	7.6	7.9	8.2	8.5	8.7	9.0	9.3	9.6	9.8	10.1	10.4	10.7	10.9
9.0	9.4	9.7	10.1	10.4	10.8	11.1	11.5	11.8	12.2	12.5	12.9	13.2	13.6	14.0
10.1	10.5	10.9	11.3	11.7	12.1	12.5	12.9	13.3	13.7	14.1	14.5	14.9	15.3	15.7
8.4	8.8	9.1	9.4	9.8	10.1	10.4	10.8	11.1	11.4	11.7	12.1	12.4	12.7	13.1
8.1	8.4	8.7	9.0	9.3	9.7	10.0	10.3	10.6	10.9	11.2	11.6	11.9	12.2	12.5
4.7	4.9	5.1	5.3	5.5	5.6	5.8	6.0	6.2	6.4	6.6	6.7	6.9	7.1	7.3

Calories Expended by Body Weight

		Your Body Weight								
Activity	**kg** **lb**	**50** **110**	**53** **117**	**56** **123**	**59** **130**	**62** **137**	**65** **143**	**68** **150**	**71** **157**	**74** **163**
Baseball										
Catcher		4.6	4.8	5.1	5.4	5.6	5.9	6.2	6.5	6.7
Infielder		4.0	4.3	4.5	4.7	5.0	5.2	5.5	5.7	6.0
Outfielder		3.9	4.1	4.3	4.5	4.8	5.0	5.2	5.5	5.7
Pitcher		4.9	5.2	5.5	5.8	6.1	6.4	6.7	7.0	7.3
Playing catch		2.2	2.3	2.5	2.6	2.7	2.8	3.0	3.1	3.2
Basketball										
Game (pickup, playground)		7.0	7.4	7.8	8.3	8.7	9.1	9.5	9.9	10.4
Game (structured, with officials)		7.4	7.9	8.3	8.8	9.2	9.7	10.1	10.6	11.0
Nongame, general shooting around		5.3	5.6	5.9	6.2	6.5	6.8	7.1	7.5	7.8
Officiating		3.9	4.2	4.4	4.6	4.9	5.1	5.4	5.6	5.8
Shooting baskets, practice		6.1	6.5	6.9	7.2	7.6	8.0	8.3	8.7	9.1
Wheelchair		5.7	6.0	6.4	6.7	7.1	7.4	7.7	8.1	8.4
Wheelchair competition, full-court game		5.7	6.0	6.3	6.7	7.0	7.3	7.7	8.0	8.4
Bathing (Sitting)		1.8	1.9	2.0	2.1	2.2	2.3	2.4	2.5	2.6
Baton Twirling		6.3	6.7	7.1	7.4	7.8	8.2	8.6	8.9	9.3
Bench Stepping										
30 step-cycles/min.; 6 in. bench		7.1	7.5	7.9	8.4	8.8	9.2	9.7	10.1	10.5
30 step-cycles/min.; 8 in. bench		7.8	8.3	8.8	9.2	9.7	10.2	10.6	11.1	11.6
30 step-cycles/min.; 10 in. bench		8.5	9.0	9.5	10.0	10.5	11.0	11.5	12.0	12.5
30 step-cycles/min.; 12 in. bench		9.3	9.9	10.4	11.0	11.6	12.1	12.7	13.2	13.8
In water, 22 step-cycles/min.; 12 in. bench		4.7	4.9	5.2	5.5	5.8	6.1	6.3	6.6	6.9
In water, 26 step-cycles/min.; 12 in. bench		5.3	5.7	6.0	6.3	6.6	6.9	7.3	7.6	7.9
In water, 28 step-cycles/min.; 12 in. bench		6.0	6.4	6.7	7.1	7.4	7.8	8.2	8.5	8.9
Bicycling—Road										
Less than 10 mph, general, leisure (cycling to work or for pleasure)		3.5	3.7	3.9	4.1	4.3	4.6	4.8	5.0	5.2
10.0–11.9 mph, leisure, slow, light effort		5.3	5.6	5.9	6.2	6.5	6.8	7.1	7.5	7.8

Calories Expended by Body Weight

Your Body Weight

77 170	80 176	83 183	86 190	89 196	92 203	95 209	98 216	101 223	104 229	107 236	110 243	113 249	116 256	119 262
7.0	7.3	7.6	7.8	8.1	8.4	8.6	8.9	9.2	9.5	9.7	10.0	10.3	10.6	10.8
6.2	6.4	6.7	6.9	7.2	7.4	7.6	7.9	8.1	8.4	8.6	8.9	9.1	9.3	9.6
5.9	6.2	6.4	6.6	6.9	7.1	7.3	7.5	7.8	8.0	8.2	8.5	8.7	8.9	9.2
7.5	7.8	8.1	8.4	8.7	9.0	9.3	9.6	9.9	10.2	10.5	10.8	11.1	11.4	11.7
3.4	3.5	3.6	3.8	3.9	4.0	4.2	4.3	4.4	4.6	4.7	4.8	4.9	5.1	5.2
10.8	11.2	11.6	12.0	12.5	12.9	13.3	13.7	14.1	14.6	15.0	15.4	15.8	16.2	16.7
11.5	11.9	12.3	12.8	13.2	13.7	14.1	14.6	15.0	15.5	15.9	16.4	16.8	17.3	17.7
8.1	8.4	8.7	9.0	9.3	9.7	10.0	10.3	10.6	10.9	11.2	11.6	11.9	12.2	12.5
6.1	6.3	6.5	6.8	7.0	7.2	7.5	7.7	8.0	8.2	8.4	8.7	8.9	9.1	9.4
9.4	9.8	10.2	10.5	10.9	11.3	11.6	12.0	12.4	12.7	13.1	13.5	13.8	14.2	14.6
8.8	9.1	9.4	9.8	10.1	10.5	10.8	11.1	11.5	11.8	12.2	12.5	12.9	13.2	13.5
8.7	9.0	9.4	9.7	10.1	10.4	10.7	11.1	11.4	11.8	12.1	12.4	12.8	13.1	13.5
2.7	2.8	2.9	3.0	3.1	3.2	3.3	3.4	3.5	3.6	3.7	3.9	4.0	4.1	4.2
9.7	10.1	10.5	10.8	11.2	11.6	12.0	12.3	12.7	13.1	13.5	13.9	14.2	14.6	15.0
10.9	11.4	11.8	12.2	12.6	13.1	13.5	13.9	14.3	14.8	15.2	15.6	16.0	16.5	16.9
12.0	12.5	13.0	13.5	13.9	14.4	14.9	15.3	15.8	16.3	16.7	17.2	17.7	18.1	18.6
13.0	13.5	14.0	14.5	15.0	15.6	16.1	16.6	17.1	17.6	18.1	18.6	19.1	19.6	20.1
14.4	14.9	15.5	16.0	16.6	17.2	17.7	18.3	18.8	19.4	20.0	20.5	21.1	21.6	22.2
7.2	7.5	7.7	8.0	8.3	8.6	8.9	9.1	9.4	9.7	10.0	10.3	10.5	10.8	11.1
8.2	8.5	8.9	9.2	9.5	9.8	10.1	10.5	10.8	11.1	11.4	11.7	12.1	12.4	12.7
9.2	9.6	10.0	10.3	10.7	11.0	11.4	11.8	12.1	12.5	12.8	13.2	13.6	13.9	14.3
5.4	5.6	5.8	6.0	6.2	6.4	6.7	6.9	7.1	7.3	7.5	7.7	7.9	8.1	8.3
8.1	8.4	8.7	9.0	9.3	9.7	10.0	10.3	10.6	10.9	11.2	11.6	11.9	12.2	12.5

Calories Expended by Body Weight

		Your Body Weight								
Activity	**kg lb**	**50 110**	**53 117**	**56 123**	**59 130**	**62 137**	**65 143**	**68 150**	**71 157**	**74 163**
Bicycling—Road (cont.)										
12.0–13.9 mph, leisure, moderate effort		7.0	7.4	7.8	8.3	8.7	9.1	9.5	9.9	10.4
14.0–15.9 mph, racing or leisure, fast, vigorous effort		8.8	9.3	9.8	10.3	10.9	11.4	11.9	12.4	13.0
16–19 mph, racing/not drafting or more than 19 mph drafting, very fast, racing		10.5	11.1	11.8	12.4	13.0	13.7	14.3	14.9	15.5
More than 19 mph, racing, no drafting		14.0	14.8	15.7	16.5	17.4	18.2	19.0	19.9	20.7
BMX or mountain trails		7.4	7.9	8.3	8.8	9.2	9.7	10.1	10.6	11.0
Bicycling—Schwinn Airdyne (Upper Extremity Mode)										
300 kg·m/min.		4.1	4.3	4.6	4.8	5.1	5.3	5.6	5.8	6.1
450 kg·m/min.		5.3	5.6	5.9	6.2	6.5	6.8	7.1	7.5	7.8
600 kg·m/min.		6.4	6.8	7.2	7.6	7.9	8.3	8.7	9.1	9.5
750 kg·m/min.		7.6	8.0	8.5	8.9	9.4	9.8	10.3	10.7	11.2
900 kg·m/min.		8.7	9.2	9.8	10.3	10.8	11.3	11.9	12.4	12.9
78% of max heart rate, arms and legs, women		6.7	7.0	7.4	7.8	8.2	8.6	9.0	9.4	9.8
78% of max heart rate, arms and legs, men		8.5	9.0	9.5	10.1	10.6	11.1	11.6	12.1	12.6
Bicycling—Stationary										
25 watts, 60 rpm, women		2.4	2.5	2.6	2.8	2.9	3.1	3.2	3.4	3.5
25 watts, 60 rpm, men		2.6	2.8	2.9	3.1	3.2	3.4	3.5	3.7	3.9
30 watts, 60 rpm		2.8	2.9	3.1	3.3	3.5	3.6	3.8	4.0	4.1
50 watts, 60 rpm, women		3.4	3.6	3.8	4.0	4.2	4.4	4.6	4.8	5.0
50 watts, 60 rpm, men		4.0	4.2	4.4	4.7	4.9	5.2	5.4	5.6	5.9
75 watts, 60 rpm, women		4.2	4.5	4.7	5.0	5.2	5.5	5.7	6.0	6.2
75 watts, 60 rpm, men		5.2	5.5	5.9	6.2	6.5	6.8	7.1	7.4	7.7
100 watts, 60 rpm, women		5.0	5.3	5.6	5.9	6.2	6.5	6.8	7.1	7.4
100 watts, 60 rpm, men		6.5	6.9	7.3	7.7	8.1	8.5	8.8	9.2	9.6
125 watts, 60 rpm, women		5.8	6.2	6.5	6.9	7.2	7.6	7.9	8.3	8.6
125 watts, 60 rpm, men		7.8	8.2	8.7	9.2	9.6	10.1	10.6	11.0	11.5
150 watts, 60 rpm, women		6.6	7.0	7.4	7.8	8.2	8.6	8.9	9.3	9.7
150 watts, 60 rpm, men		9.0	9.6	10.1	10.7	11.2	11.7	12.3	12.8	13.4
175 watts, 60 rpm, women		7.4	7.8	8.3	8.7	9.1	9.6	10.0	10.5	10.9

Calories Expended by Body Weight

Your Body Weight

77	80	83	86	89	92	95	98	101	104	107	110	113	116	119
170	176	183	190	196	203	209	216	223	229	236	243	249	256	262

10.8	11.2	11.6	12.0	12.5	12.9	13.3	13.7	14.1	14.6	15.0	15.4	15.8	16.2	16.7
13.5	14.0	14.5	15.1	15.6	16.1	16.6	17.2	17.7	18.2	18.7	19.3	19.8	20.3	20.8
16.2	16.8	17.4	18.1	18.7	19.3	20.0	20.6	21.2	21.8	22.5	23.1	23.7	24.4	25.0
21.6	22.4	23.2	24.1	24.9	25.8	26.6	27.4	28.3	29.1	30.0	30.8	31.6	32.5	33.3
11.5	11.9	12.3	12.8	13.2	13.7	14.1	14.6	15.0	15.5	15.9	16.4	16.8	17.3	17.7

6.3	6.6	6.8	7.0	7.3	7.5	7.8	8.0	8.3	8.5	8.8	9.0	9.3	9.5	9.7
8.1	8.4	8.7	9.0	9.3	9.7	10.0	10.3	10.6	10.9	11.2	11.6	11.9	12.2	12.5
9.9	10.2	10.6	11.0	11.4	11.8	12.2	12.6	12.9	13.3	13.7	14.1	14.5	14.9	15.2
11.6	12.1	12.5	13.0	13.5	13.9	14.4	14.8	15.3	15.7	16.2	16.6	17.1	17.5	18.0
13.4	13.9	14.5	15.0	15.5	16.0	16.6	17.1	17.6	18.1	18.7	19.2	19.7	20.2	20.7
10.2	10.6	11.0	11.4	11.8	12.2	12.6	13.0	13.4	13.8	14.2	14.6	15.0	15.4	15.8
13.1	13.6	14.1	14.7	15.2	15.7	16.2	16.7	17.2	17.7	18.2	18.7	19.3	19.8	20.3

3.6	3.8	3.9	4.1	4.2	4.3	4.5	4.6	4.8	4.9	5.1	5.2	5.3	5.5	5.6
4.0	4.2	4.3	4.5	4.6	4.8	5.0	5.1	5.3	5.4	5.6	5.7	5.9	6.0	6.2
4.3	4.5	4.6	4.8	5.0	5.1	5.3	5.5	5.6	5.8	6.0	6.1	6.3	6.5	6.6
5.2	5.4	5.7	5.9	6.1	6.3	6.5	6.7	6.9	7.1	7.3	7.5	7.7	7.9	8.1
6.1	6.4	6.6	6.8	7.1	7.3	7.5	7.8	8.0	8.3	8.5	8.7	9.0	9.2	9.5
6.5	6.7	7.0	7.2	7.5	7.7	8.0	8.2	8.5	8.7	9.0	9.2	9.5	9.7	10.0
8.1	8.4	8.7	9.0	9.3	9.6	9.9	10.3	10.6	10.9	11.2	11.5	11.8	12.1	12.5
7.7	8.0	8.3	8.6	8.9	9.2	9.5	9.8	10.1	10.4	10.7	11.0	11.3	11.6	11.9
10.0	10.4	10.8	11.2	11.6	12.0	12.4	12.7	13.1	13.5	13.9	14.3	14.7	15.1	15.5
9.0	9.3	9.7	10.0	10.4	10.7	11.1	11.4	11.8	12.1	12.5	12.8	13.2	13.5	13.9
12.0	12.4	12.9	13.3	13.8	14.3	14.7	15.2	15.7	16.1	16.6	17.1	17.5	18.0	18.5
10.1	10.5	10.9	11.3	11.7	12.1	12.5	12.9	13.3	13.7	14.1	14.5	14.9	15.3	15.7
13.9	14.4	15.0	15.5	16.1	16.6	17.2	17.7	18.2	18.8	19.3	19.9	20.4	20.9	21.5
11.4	11.8	12.2	12.7	13.1	13.6	14.0	14.5	14.9	15.3	15.8	16.2	16.7	17.1	17.6

Calories Expended by Body Weight

		Your Body Weight								
Activity	**kg** **lb**	**50** **110**	**53** **117**	**56** **123**	**59** **130**	**62** **137**	**65** **143**	**68** **150**	**71** **157**	**74** **163**
Bicycling—Stationary (cont.)										
175 watts, 60 rpm, men		10.3	10.9	11.5	12.1	12.8	13.4	14.0	14.6	15.2
200 watts, 60 rpm, women		8.2	8.7	9.2	9.6	10.1	10.6	11.1	11.6	12.1
200 watts, 60 rpm, men		11.6	12.3	12.9	13.6	14.3	15.0	15.7	16.4	17.1
200 watts, 50, 65, 80 rpm, Schwinn Velodyne Trainer		10.6	11.2	11.9	12.5	13.1	13.8	14.4	15.0	15.7
200 watts, 90 rpm, Schwinn Velodyne Trainer		11.4	12.1	12.7	13.4	14.1	14.8	15.5	16.2	16.8
200 watts, 110 rpm, Schwinn Velodyne Trainer		12.0	12.7	13.4	14.2	14.9	15.6	16.3	17.0	17.8
Pregnant 25 wk; Tunturi semirecumbent, (135–140 beats/min.)		4.9	5.2	5.5	5.8	6.1	6.4	6.7	7.0	7.3
Billiards		2.2	2.3	2.5	2.6	2.7	2.8	3.0	3.1	3.2
Boating (Power)		2.2	2.3	2.5	2.6	2.7	2.8	3.0	3.1	3.2
Bookbinding		2.0	2.1	2.3	2.4	2.5	2.6	2.7	2.9	3.0
Bowling		2.6	2.8	2.9	3.1	3.3	3.4	3.6	3.7	3.9
Boxing										
Competition in ring		11.4	12.1	12.7	13.4	14.1	14.8	15.5	16.2	16.8
Punching bag, fast bag		6.3	6.7	7.1	7.4	7.8	8.2	8.6	8.9	9.3
Shadow boxing		5.3	5.6	5.9	6.2	6.5	6.8	7.1	7.5	7.8
Sparring in ring with opponent		7.9	8.3	8.8	9.3	9.8	10.2	10.7	11.2	11.7
Broomball		6.1	6.5	6.9	7.2	7.6	8.0	8.3	8.7	9.1
Building Road										
Directing traffic (standing)		1.8	1.9	2.0	2.1	2.2	2.3	2.4	2.5	2.6
Hauling debris, driving heavy machinery		5.3	5.6	5.9	6.2	6.5	6.8	7.1	7.5	7.8
Calisthenics										
Home exercise, light or moderate effort, general		3.9	4.2	4.4	4.6	4.9	5.1	5.4	5.6	5.8
Performed vigorously (push-ups, pull-ups, sit-ups)		7.0	7.4	7.8	8.3	8.7	9.1	9.5	9.9	10.4

Calories Expended by Body Weight

Your Body Weight

77	80	83	86	89	92	95	98	101	104	107	110	113	116	119
170	176	183	190	196	203	209	216	223	229	236	243	249	256	262
15.8	16.5	17.1	17.7	18.3	18.9	19.6	20.2	20.8	21.4	22.0	22.6	23.3	23.9	24.5
12.6	13.1	13.6	14.1	14.5	15.0	15.5	16.0	16.5	17.0	17.5	18.0	18.5	19.0	19.5
17.8	18.5	19.2	19.9	20.6	21.3	22.0	22.7	23.3	24.0	24.7	25.4	26.1	26.8	27.5
16.3	16.9	17.6	18.2	18.8	19.5	20.1	20.8	21.4	22.0	22.7	23.3	23.9	24.6	25.2
17.5	18.2	18.9	19.6	20.2	20.9	21.6	22.3	23.0	23.7	24.3	25.0	25.7	26.4	27.1
18.5	19.2	19.9	20.6	21.4	22.1	22.8	23.5	24.2	25.0	25.7	26.4	27.1	27.8	28.6
7.6	7.9	8.2	8.5	8.8	9.1	9.4	9.7	10.0	10.3	10.6	10.9	11.2	11.5	11.8
3.4	3.5	3.6	3.8	3.9	4.0	4.2	4.3	4.4	4.6	4.7	4.8	4.9	5.1	5.2
3.4	3.5	3.6	3.8	3.9	4.0	4.2	4.3	4.4	4.6	4.7	4.8	4.9	5.1	5.2
3.1	3.2	3.3	3.5	3.6	3.7	3.8	3.9	4.1	4.2	4.3	4.4	4.5	4.7	4.8
4.0	4.2	4.4	4.5	4.7	4.8	5.0	5.1	5.3	5.5	5.6	5.8	5.9	6.1	6.2
17.5	18.2	18.9	19.6	20.2	20.9	21.6	22.3	23.0	23.7	24.3	25.0	25.7	26.4	27.1
9.7	10.1	10.5	10.8	11.2	11.6	12.0	12.3	12.7	13.1	13.5	13.9	14.2	14.6	15.0
8.1	8.4	8.7	9.0	9.3	9.7	10.0	10.3	10.6	10.9	11.2	11.6	11.9	12.2	12.5
12.1	12.6	13.1	13.5	14.0	14.5	15.0	15.4	15.9	16.4	16.9	17.3	17.8	18.3	18.7
9.4	9.8	10.2	10.5	10.9	11.3	11.6	12.0	12.4	12.7	13.1	13.5	13.8	14.2	14.6
2.7	2.8	2.9	3.0	3.1	3.2	3.3	3.4	3.5	3.6	3.7	3.9	4.0	4.1	4.2
8.1	8.4	8.7	9.0	9.3	9.7	10.0	10.3	10.6	10.9	11.2	11.6	11.9	12.2	12.5
6.1	6.3	6.5	6.8	7.0	7.2	7.5	7.7	8.0	8.2	8.4	8.7	8.9	9.1	9.4
10.8	11.2	11.6	12.0	12.5	12.9	13.3	13.7	14.1	14.6	15.0	15.4	15.8	16.2	16.7

Calories Expended by Body Weight

Activity	kg lb	50 110	53 117	56 123	59 130	62 137	65 143	68 150	71 157	74 163
Calisthenics (cont.)										
Stretching, general		3.5	3.7	3.9	4.1	4.3	4.6	4.8	5.0	5.2
Water calisthenics		3.5	3.7	3.9	4.1	4.3	4.6	4.8	5.0	5.2
Canadian Aerobic Fitness Test (Step-Test)										
Level 1: 8 in. bench, 4 steps/cycle		4.0	4.2	4.5	4.7	5.0	5.2	5.4	5.7	5.9
Level 2: 8 in. bench, 4 steps/cycle		4.5	4.8	5.1	5.3	5.6	5.9	6.2	6.4	6.7
Level 3: 8 in. bench, 4 steps/cycle		5.5	5.8	6.2	6.5	6.8	7.2	7.5	7.8	8.1
Level 4: 8 in. bench, 4 steps/cycle		6.2	6.5	6.9	7.3	7.6	8.0	8.4	8.7	9.1
Level 5: 8 in. bench, 4 steps/cycle		7.1	7.5	7.9	8.4	8.8	9.2	9.6	10.1	10.5
Level 6: 8 in. bench, 4 steps/cycle		8.0	8.5	9.0	9.4	9.9	10.4	10.9	11.4	11.8
Level 7: 16 in. bench, 4 steps/cycle		8.8	9.3	9.8	10.4	10.9	11.4	11.9	12.5	13.0
Level 8: 16 in. bench, 4 steps/cycle		9.9	10.4	11.0	11.6	12.2	12.8	13.4	14.0	14.6
Canoeing										
2.0–3.9 mph, light effort		2.6	2.8	2.9	3.1	3.3	3.4	3.6	3.7	3.9
4.0–5.9 mph, moderate effort		6.1	6.5	6.9	7.2	7.6	8.0	8.3	8.7	9.1
More than 5.9 mph, vigorous effort		10.5	11.1	11.8	12.4	13.0	13.7	14.3	14.9	15.5
Camping trip		3.5	3.7	3.9	4.1	4.3	4.6	4.8	5.0	5.2
Competition, crew or sculling		10.5	11.1	11.8	12.4	13.0	13.7	14.3	14.9	15.5
Pleasure, general		3.1	3.2	3.4	3.6	3.8	4.0	4.2	4.3	4.5
Portaging		6.1	6.5	6.9	7.2	7.6	8.0	8.3	8.7	9.1
White water (recreational)		4.4	4.6	4.9	5.2	5.4	5.7	6.0	6.2	6.5
Cardiopulmonary Resuscitation (CPR)										
Compressor role		2.8	3.0	3.1	3.3	3.5	3.6	3.8	4.0	4.1
Ventilator role		1.5	1.6	1.7	1.8	1.8	1.9	2.0	2.1	2.2
One-person		3.4	3.6	3.8	4.0	4.2	4.4	4.6	4.8	5.1
Carpentry										
Finishing or refinishing cabinets or furniture		3.9	4.2	4.4	4.6	4.9	5.1	5.4	5.6	5.8
General		3.1	3.2	3.4	3.6	3.8	4.0	4.2	4.3	4.5
General, workshop (standing)		2.6	2.8	2.9	3.1	3.3	3.4	3.6	3.7	3.9
Outside house, installing gutters, windows, building decks		5.3	5.6	5.9	6.2	6.5	6.8	7.1	7.5	7.8
Sawing hardwood		6.6	7.0	7.4	7.7	8.1	8.5	8.9	9.3	9.7

Calories Expended by Body Weight

Your Body Weight

77 170	80 176	83 183	86 190	89 196	92 203	95 209	98 216	101 223	104 229	107 236	110 243	113 249	116 256	119 262
5.4	5.6	5.8	6.0	6.2	6.4	6.7	6.9	7.1	7.3	7.5	7.7	7.9	8.1	8.3
5.4	5.6	5.8	6.0	6.2	6.4	6.7	6.9	7.1	7.3	7.5	7.7	7.9	8.1	8.3
6.2	6.4	6.6	6.9	7.1	7.4	7.6	7.8	8.1	8.3	8.6	8.8	9.0	9.3	9.5
7.0	7.2	7.5	7.8	8.1	8.3	8.6	8.9	9.1	9.4	9.7	10.0	10.2	10.5	10.8
8.5	8.8	9.1	9.5	9.8	10.1	10.5	10.8	11.1	11.4	11.8	12.1	12.4	12.8	13.1
9.5	9.8	10.2	10.6	10.9	11.3	11.7	12.1	12.4	12.8	13.2	13.5	13.9	14.3	14.6
10.9	11.3	11.8	12.2	12.6	13.0	13.4	13.9	14.3	14.7	15.1	15.6	16.0	16.4	16.8
12.3	12.8	13.3	13.8	14.2	14.7	15.2	15.7	16.2	16.6	17.1	17.6	18.1	18.6	19.0
13.5	14.0	14.6	15.1	15.6	16.1	16.7	17.2	17.7	18.3	18.8	19.3	19.8	20.4	20.9
15.2	15.8	16.4	16.9	17.5	18.1	18.7	19.3	19.9	20.5	21.1	21.7	22.3	22.9	23.4
4.0	4.2	4.4	4.5	4.7	4.8	5.0	5.1	5.3	5.5	5.6	5.8	5.9	6.1	6.2
9.4	9.8	10.2	10.5	10.9	11.3	11.6	12.0	12.4	12.7	13.1	13.5	13.8	14.2	14.6
16.2	16.8	17.4	18.1	18.7	19.3	20.0	20.6	21.2	21.8	22.5	23.1	23.7	24.4	25.0
5.4	5.6	5.8	6.0	6.2	6.4	6.7	6.9	7.1	7.3	7.5	7.7	7.9	8.1	8.3
16.2	16.8	17.4	18.1	18.7	19.3	20.0	20.6	21.2	21.8	22.5	23.1	23.7	24.4	25.0
4.7	4.9	5.1	5.3	5.5	5.6	5.8	6.0	6.2	6.4	6.6	6.7	6.9	7.1	7.3
9.4	9.8	10.2	10.5	10.9	11.3	11.6	12.0	12.4	12.7	13.1	13.5	13.8	14.2	14.6
6.7	7.0	7.3	7.5	7.8	8.1	8.3	8.6	8.8	9.1	9.4	9.6	9.9	10.2	10.4
4.3	4.5	4.6	4.8	5.0	5.2	5.3	5.5	5.7	5.8	6.0	6.2	6.3	6.5	6.7
2.3	2.4	2.5	2.6	2.6	2.7	2.8	2.9	3.0	3.1	3.2	3.3	3.4	3.5	3.5
5.3	5.5	5.7	5.9	6.1	6.3	6.5	6.7	6.9	7.1	7.3	7.5	7.7	7.9	8.1
6.1	6.3	6.5	6.8	7.0	7.2	7.5	7.7	8.0	8.2	8.4	8.7	8.9	9.1	9.4
4.7	4.9	5.1	5.3	5.5	5.6	5.8	6.0	6.2	6.4	6.6	6.7	6.9	7.1	7.3
4.0	4.2	4.4	4.5	4.7	4.8	5.0	5.1	5.3	5.5	5.6	5.8	5.9	6.1	6.2
8.1	8.4	8.7	9.0	9.3	9.7	10.0	10.3	10.6	10.9	11.2	11.6	11.9	12.2	12.5
10.1	10.5	10.9	11.3	11.7	12.1	12.5	12.9	13.3	13.7	14.0	14.4	14.8	15.2	15.6

Calories Expended by Body Weight

						Your Body Weight				
Activity	**kg** **lb**	**50** **110**	**53** **117**	**56** **123**	**59** **130**	**62** **137**	**65** **143**	**68** **150**	**71** **157**	**74** **163**
Carpet Sweeping— *Sweeping Floors*		2.2	2.3	2.5	2.6	2.7	2.8	3.0	3.1	3.2
Carrying Loads										
1–15 lb load, up stairs		4.4	4.6	4.9	5.2	5.4	5.7	6.0	6.2	6.5
16–24 lb load, up stairs		5.3	5.6	5.9	6.2	6.5	6.8	7.1	7.5	7.8
25–49 lb load, up stairs		7.0	7.4	7.8	8.3	8.7	9.1	9.5	9.9	10.4
50–74 lb load, up stairs		8.8	9.3	9.8	10.3	10.9	11.4	11.9	12.4	13.0
More than 74 lb load, up stairs		10.5	11.1	11.8	12.4	13.0	13.7	14.3	14.9	15.5
Groceries		7.0	7.4	7.8	8.3	8.7	9.1	9.5	9.9	10.4
Heavy loads (bricks, lumber)		7.0	7.4	7.8	8.3	8.7	9.1	9.5	9.9	10.4
Infant or 15 lb load (suitcase), level ground or down stairs		3.1	3.2	3.4	3.6	3.8	4.0	4.2	4.3	4.5
Lumber (carrying, loading/ unloading, stacking)		4.4	4.6	4.9	5.2	5.4	5.7	6.0	6.2	6.5
Moderate loads up stairs, (16–40 lb)		7.0	7.4	7.8	8.3	8.7	9.1	9.5	9.9	10.4
Upstairs, general		7.9	8.3	8.8	9.3	9.8	10.2	10.7	11.2	11.7
Caulking										
Chinking log cabin		4.4	4.6	4.9	5.2	5.4	5.7	6.0	6.2	6.5
General		3.9	4.2	4.4	4.6	4.9	5.1	5.4	5.6	5.8
Cello Playing		1.8	1.9	2.0	2.1	2.2	2.3	2.4	2.5	2.6
Chambermaid		2.2	2.3	2.5	2.6	2.7	2.8	3.0	3.1	3.2
Child Care										
Games (hopscotch, 4-square, dodgeball, playground, T-ball, kick the can, tetherball, marbles, jacks, arcade games)		4.4	4.6	4.9	5.2	5.4	5.7	6.0	6.2	6.5
Pushing or pulling child in stroller, walking		2.2	2.3	2.5	2.6	2.7	2.8	3.0	3.1	3.2
Sitting/kneeling (dressing, bathing, grooming, feeding, occasional lifting of child, light effort)		2.6	2.8	2.9	3.1	3.3	3.4	3.6	3.7	3.9
Standing (dressing, bathing, grooming, feeding, occasional lifting of child, light effort)		3.1	3.2	3.4	3.6	3.8	4.0	4.2	4.3	4.5

Calories Expended by Body Weight

Your Body Weight

77 170	80 176	83 183	86 190	89 196	92 203	95 209	98 216	101 223	104 229	107 236	110 243	113 249	116 256	119 262
3.4	3.5	3.6	3.8	3.9	4.0	4.2	4.3	4.4	4.6	4.7	4.8	4.9	5.1	5.2
6.7	7.0	7.3	7.5	7.8	8.1	8.3	8.6	8.8	9.1	9.4	9.6	9.9	10.2	10.4
8.1	8.4	8.7	9.0	9.3	9.7	10.0	10.3	10.6	10.9	11.2	11.6	11.9	12.2	12.5
10.8	11.2	11.6	12.0	12.5	12.9	13.3	13.7	14.1	14.6	15.0	15.4	15.8	16.2	16.7
13.5	14.0	14.5	15.1	15.6	16.1	16.6	17.2	17.7	18.2	18.7	19.3	19.8	20.3	20.8
16.2	16.8	17.4	18.1	18.7	19.3	20.0	20.6	21.2	21.8	22.5	23.1	23.7	24.4	25.0
10.8	11.2	11.6	12.0	12.5	12.9	13.3	13.7	14.1	14.6	15.0	15.4	15.8	16.2	16.7
10.8	11.2	11.6	12.0	12.5	12.9	13.3	13.7	14.1	14.6	15.0	15.4	15.8	16.2	16.7
4.7	4.9	5.1	5.3	5.5	5.6	5.8	6.0	6.2	6.4	6.6	6.7	6.9	7.1	7.3
6.7	7.0	7.3	7.5	7.8	8.1	8.3	8.6	8.8	9.1	9.4	9.6	9.9	10.2	10.4
10.8	11.2	11.6	12.0	12.5	12.9	13.3	13.7	14.1	14.6	15.0	15.4	15.8	16.2	16.7
12.1	12.6	13.1	13.5	14.0	14.5	15.0	15.4	15.9	16.4	16.9	17.3	17.8	18.3	18.7
6.7	7.0	7.3	7.5	7.8	8.1	8.3	8.6	8.8	9.1	9.4	9.6	9.9	10.2	10.4
6.1	6.3	6.5	6.8	7.0	7.2	7.5	7.7	8.0	8.2	8.4	8.7	8.9	9.1	9.4
2.7	2.8	2.9	3.0	3.1	3.2	3.3	3.4	3.5	3.6	3.7	3.9	4.0	4.1	4.2
3.4	3.5	3.6	3.8	3.9	4.0	4.2	4.3	4.4	4.6	4.7	4.8	4.9	5.1	5.2
6.7	7.0	7.3	7.5	7.8	8.1	8.3	8.6	8.8	9.1	9.4	9.6	9.9	10.2	10.4
3.4	3.5	3.6	3.8	3.9	4.0	4.2	4.3	4.4	4.6	4.7	4.8	4.9	5.1	5.2
4.0	4.2	4.4	4.5	4.7	4.8	5.0	5.1	5.3	5.5	5.6	5.8	5.9	6.1	6.2
4.7	4.9	5.1	5.3	5.5	5.6	5.8	6.0	6.2	6.4	6.6	6.7	6.9	7.1	7.3

Calories Expended by Body Weight

					Your Body Weight					
Activity	**kg** **lb**	**50** **110**	**53** **117**	**56** **123**	**59** **130**	**62** **137**	**65** **143**	**68** **150**	**71** **157**	**74** **163**
Child Care (cont.)										
Walk/run-playing with child, vigorous		4.4	4.6	4.9	5.2	5.4	5.7	6.0	6.2	6.5
Walk/run-playing with child, moderate		3.5	3.7	3.9	4.1	4.3	4.6	4.8	5.0	5.2
Chopping Wood—Splitting Logs		5.3	5.6	5.9	6.2	6.5	6.8	7.1	7.5	7.8
Cleaning										
Gutters, scrubbing decks		4.4	4.6	4.9	5.2	5.4	5.7	6.0	6.2	6.5
Heavy, continuous effort (washing car, washing windows, mopping, cleaning garage)		3.9	4.2	4.4	4.6	4.9	5.1	5.4	5.6	5.8
Home, general		3.1	3.2	3.4	3.6	3.8	4.0	4.2	4.3	4.5
Light (dusting, straightening up, vacuuming, changing linen, carrying out trash)		2.2	2.3	2.5	2.6	2.7	2.8	3.0	3.1	3.2
Walking, moderate effort (putting away household items)		2.6	2.8	2.9	3.1	3.3	3.4	3.6	3.7	3.9
Clearing Land— Hauling Branches		4.4	4.6	4.9	5.2	5.4	5.7	6.0	6.2	6.5
Climbing Hills										
0–9 lb load		6.1	6.5	6.9	7.2	7.6	8.0	8.3	8.7	9.1
10 to 20 lb load		6.6	7.0	7.4	7.7	8.1	8.5	8.9	9.3	9.7
21 to 42 lb load		7.0	7.4	7.8	8.3	8.7	9.1	9.5	9.9	10.4
More than 42 lb load		7.9	8.3	8.8	9.3	9.8	10.2	10.7	11.2	11.7
Coaching										
Football, soccer, basketball, baseball, swimming, lacrosse, softball, track		3.5	3.7	3.9	4.1	4.3	4.6	4.8	5.0	5.2
Coal Mining										
Drilling coal, rock		5.7	6.0	6.4	6.7	7.1	7.4	7.7	8.1	8.4
Erecting supports		5.7	6.0	6.4	6.7	7.1	7.4	7.7	8.1	8.4
General		5.3	5.6	5.9	6.2	6.5	6.8	7.1	7.5	7.8
Shoveling coal		6.1	6.5	6.9	7.2	7.6	8.0	8.3	8.7	9.1

Calories Expended by Body Weight

Your Body Weight

77 170	80 176	83 183	86 190	89 196	92 203	95 209	98 216	101 223	104 229	107 236	110 243	113 249	116 256	119 262
6.7	7.0	7.3	7.5	7.8	8.1	8.3	8.6	8.8	9.1	9.4	9.6	9.9	10.2	10.4
5.4	5.6	5.8	6.0	6.2	6.4	6.7	6.9	7.1	7.3	7.5	7.7	7.9	8.1	8.3
8.1	8.4	8.7	9.0	9.3	9.7	10.0	10.3	10.6	10.9	11.2	11.6	11.9	12.2	12.5
6.7	7.0	7.3	7.5	7.8	8.1	8.3	8.6	8.8	9.1	9.4	9.6	9.9	10.2	10.4
6.1	6.3	6.5	6.8	7.0	7.2	7.5	7.7	8.0	8.2	8.4	8.7	8.9	9.1	9.4
4.7	4.9	5.1	5.3	5.5	5.6	5.8	6.0	6.2	6.4	6.6	6.7	6.9	7.1	7.3
3.4	3.5	3.6	3.8	3.9	4.0	4.2	4.3	4.4	4.6	4.7	4.8	4.9	5.1	5.2
4.0	4.2	4.4	4.5	4.7	4.8	5.0	5.1	5.3	5.5	5.6	5.8	5.9	6.1	6.2
6.7	7.0	7.3	7.5	7.8	8.1	8.3	8.6	8.8	9.1	9.4	9.6	9.9	10.2	10.4
9.4	9.8	10.2	10.5	10.9	11.3	11.6	12.0	12.4	12.7	13.1	13.5	13.8	14.2	14.6
10.1	10.5	10.9	11.3	11.7	12.1	12.5	12.9	13.3	13.7	14.0	14.4	14.8	15.2	15.6
10.8	11.2	11.6	12.0	12.5	12.9	13.3	13.7	14.1	14.6	15.0	15.4	15.8	16.2	16.7
12.1	12.6	13.1	13.5	14.0	14.5	15.0	15.4	15.9	16.4	16.9	17.3	17.8	18.3	18.7
5.4	5.6	5.8	6.0	6.2	6.4	6.7	6.9	7.1	7.3	7.5	7.7	7.9	8.1	8.3
8.8	9.1	9.4	9.8	10.1	10.5	10.8	11.1	11.5	11.8	12.2	12.5	12.9	13.2	13.5
8.8	9.1	9.4	9.8	10.1	10.5	10.8	11.1	11.5	11.8	12.2	12.5	12.9	13.2	13.5
8.1	8.4	8.7	9.0	9.3	9.7	10.0	10.3	10.6	10.9	11.2	11.6	11.9	12.2	12.5
9.4	9.8	10.2	10.5	10.9	11.3	11.6	12.0	12.4	12.7	13.1	13.5	13.8	14.2	14.6

Calories Expended by Body Weight

Your Body Weight

Activity	kg 50 lb 110	53 117	56 123	59 130	62 137	65 143	68 150	71 157	74 163
Conducting Orchestra, Chorus	2.2	2.3	2.5	2.6	2.7	2.8	3.0	3.1	3.2
Construction									
Excavation work	4.4	4.6	4.9	5.2	5.4	5.7	6.0	6.2	6.5
Remodeling, outside	4.8	5.1	5.4	5.7	6.0	6.3	6.5	6.8	7.1
Cooking/Food Preparation and Service									
Standing, sitting, walking	2.2	2.3	2.5	2.6	2.7	2.8	3.0	3.1	3.2
Serving food, setting table, walking or standing	2.2	2.3	2.5	2.6	2.7	2.8	3.0	3.1	3.2
Cricket (Batting, Bowling, Fielding)	4.4	4.6	4.9	5.2	5.4	5.7	6.0	6.2	6.5
Croquet	2.2	2.3	2.5	2.6	2.7	2.8	3.0	3.1	3.2
Curling	6.3	6.7	7.1	7.4	7.8	8.2	8.6	8.9	9.3
Cybex UBE (Upper Body Exercise)									
400 kg·m/min., women	2.4	2.5	2.7	2.8	3.0	3.1	3.2	3.4	3.5
400 kg·m/min., men	2.6	2.8	2.9	3.1	3.2	3.4	3.5	3.7	3.8
450 kg·m/min., 30 rpm	4.1	4.3	4.6	4.8	5.0	5.3	5.5	5.8	6.0
450 kg·m/min., 60 rpm	2.9	3.1	3.2	3.4	3.6	3.7	3.9	4.1	4.3
450 kg·m/min., 90 rpm	2.0	2.2	2.3	2.4	2.5	2.7	2.8	2.9	3.0
500 kg·m/min., women	3.2	3.4	3.6	3.8	4.0	4.2	4.4	4.6	4.8
500 kg·m/min., men	3.3	3.5	3.7	3.9	4.1	4.3	4.5	4.7	4.9
600 kg·m/min., women	4.1	4.3	4.5	4.8	5.0	5.3	5.5	5.8	6.0
600 kg·m/min., men	4.1	4.3	4.6	4.8	5.1	5.3	5.6	5.8	6.0
600 kg·m/min., 30 rpm	6.2	6.6	6.9	7.3	7.7	8.1	8.4	8.8	9.2
600 kg·m/min., 60 rpm	4.0	4.2	4.5	4.7	4.9	5.2	5.4	5.7	5.9
600 kg·m/min., 90 rpm	3.2	3.4	3.6	3.8	4.0	4.2	4.4	4.5	4.7
700 kg·m/min., women	4.8	5.1	5.4	5.7	6.0	6.3	6.6	6.9	7.1
700 kg·m/min., men	4.9	5.2	5.5	5.8	6.1	6.4	6.7	6.9	7.2
750 kg·m/min., 30 rpm	8.3	8.7	9.2	9.7	10.2	10.7	11.2	11.7	12.2
750 kg·m/min., 60 rpm	4.9	5.2	5.4	5.7	6.0	6.3	6.6	6.9	7.2
750 kg·m/min., 90 rpm	4.8	5.1	5.4	5.7	6.0	6.3	6.5	6.8	7.1
800 kg·m/min., women	5.6	5.9	6.3	6.6	6.9	7.3	7.6	7.9	8.3
800 kg·m/min., men	5.7	6.1	6.4	6.8	7.1	7.5	7.8	8.1	8.5
900 kg·m/min., women	6.3	6.7	7.1	7.5	7.8	8.2	8.6	9.0	9.4
900 kg·m/min., men	6.6	7.0	7.4	7.8	8.1	8.5	8.9	9.3	9.7

Calories Expended by Body Weight

Your Body Weight

77 170	80 176	83 183	86 190	89 196	92 203	95 209	98 216	101 223	104 229	107 236	110 243	113 249	116 256	119 262
3.4	3.5	3.6	3.8	3.9	4.0	4.2	4.3	4.4	4.6	4.7	4.8	4.9	5.1	5.2
6.7	7.0	7.3	7.5	7.8	8.1	8.3	8.6	8.8	9.1	9.4	9.6	9.9	10.2	10.4
7.4	7.7	8.0	8.3	8.6	8.9	9.1	9.4	9.7	10.0	10.3	10.6	10.9	11.2	11.5
3.4	3.5	3.6	3.8	3.9	4.0	4.2	4.3	4.4	4.6	4.7	4.8	4.9	5.1	5.2
3.4	3.5	3.6	3.8	3.9	4.0	4.2	4.3	4.4	4.6	4.7	4.8	4.9	5.1	5.2
6.7	7.0	7.3	7.5	7.8	8.1	8.3	8.6	8.8	9.1	9.4	9.6	9.9	10.2	10.4
3.4	3.5	3.6	3.8	3.9	4.0	4.2	4.3	4.4	4.6	4.7	4.8	4.9	5.1	5.2
9.7	10.1	10.5	10.8	11.2	11.6	12.0	12.3	12.7	13.1	13.5	13.9	14.2	14.6	15.0
3.7	3.8	4.0	4.1	4.2	4.4	4.5	4.7	4.8	5.0	5.1	5.2	5.4	5.5	5.7
4.0	4.2	4.3	4.5	4.6	4.8	4.9	5.1	5.2	5.4	5.6	5.7	5.9	6.0	6.2
6.3	6.5	6.8	7.0	7.2	7.5	7.7	8.0	8.2	8.5	8.7	9.0	9.2	9.4	9.7
4.4	4.6	4.8	5.0	5.1	5.3	5.5	5.6	5.8	6.0	6.2	6.3	6.5	6.7	6.9
3.1	3.3	3.4	3.5	3.6	3.8	3.9	4.0	4.1	4.2	4.4	4.5	4.6	4.7	4.9
5.0	5.2	5.3	5.5	5.7	5.9	6.1	6.3	6.5	6.7	6.9	7.1	7.3	7.5	7.7
5.1	5.3	5.5	5.7	5.9	6.2	6.4	6.6	6.8	7.0	7.2	7.4	7.6	7.8	8.0
6.2	6.5	6.7	7.0	7.2	7.5	7.7	7.9	8.2	8.4	8.7	8.9	9.2	9.4	9.6
6.3	6.5	6.8	7.0	7.3	7.5	7.8	8.0	8.3	8.5	8.7	9.0	9.2	9.5	9.7
9.6	9.9	10.3	10.7	11.0	11.4	11.8	12.2	12.5	12.9	13.3	13.6	14.0	14.4	14.8
6.1	6.4	6.6	6.8	7.1	7.3	7.6	7.8	8.0	8.3	8.5	8.8	9.0	9.2	9.5
4.9	5.1	5.3	5.5	5.7	5.9	6.1	6.3	6.5	6.7	6.9	7.0	7.2	7.4	7.6
7.4	7.7	8.0	8.3	8.6	8.9	9.2	9.5	9.8	10.0	10.3	10.6	10.9	11.2	11.5
7.5	7.8	8.1	8.4	8.7	9.0	9.3	9.6	9.9	10.2	10.5	10.8	11.1	11.3	11.6
12.7	13.2	13.7	14.2	14.7	15.2	15.7	16.2	16.7	17.2	17.7	18.2	18.6	19.1	19.6
7.5	7.8	8.1	8.4	8.7	9.0	9.2	9.5	9.8	10.1	10.4	10.7	11.0	11.3	11.6
7.4	7.7	8.0	8.3	8.6	8.9	9.1	9.4	9.7	10.0	10.3	10.6	10.9	11.2	11.5
8.6	8.9	9.3	9.6	9.9	10.3	10.6	10.9	11.3	11.6	11.9	12.3	12.6	13.0	13.3
8.8	9.2	9.5	9.9	10.2	10.5	10.9	11.2	11.6	11.9	12.3	12.6	13.0	13.3	13.6
9.7	10.1	10.5	10.9	11.3	11.6	12.0	12.4	12.8	13.2	13.5	13.9	14.3	14.7	15.1
10.1	10.5	10.9	11.3	11.7	12.1	12.5	12.9	13.3	13.7	14.1	14.5	14.9	15.2	15.6

Calories Expended by Body Weight

Activity	kg lb	50 110	53 117	56 123	59 130	62 137	65 143	68 150	71 157	74 163
Cybex UBE (Upper Body Exercise) (cont.)										
1000 kg·m/min., women		7.1	7.5	7.9	8.4	8.8	9.2	9.6	10.1	10.5
1000 kg·m/min., men		7.4	7.8	8.3	8.7	9.2	9.6	10.1	10.5	11.0
Dance										
Belly-dancing routine		5.3	5.6	5.9	6.3	6.6	6.9	7.2	7.5	7.8
General (ballet, modern, swing, twist, lambada)		5.3	5.6	5.9	6.2	6.5	6.8	7.1	7.5	7.8
General (big band, rock 'n'roll)		4.2	4.5	4.7	5.0	5.2	5.5	5.7	6.0	6.2
Darts (Wall or Lawn)		2.2	2.3	2.5	2.6	2.7	2.8	3.0	3.1	3.2
Digging										
Sandbox		4.4	4.6	4.9	5.2	5.4	5.7	6.0	6.2	6.5
Spading, filling garden		4.4	4.6	4.9	5.2	5.4	5.7	6.0	6.2	6.5
Worms, with shovel		3.5	3.7	3.9	4.1	4.3	4.6	4.8	5.0	5.2
Diving (Springboard or Platform)		2.6	2.8	2.9	3.1	3.3	3.4	3.6	3.7	3.9
Dressing/Undressing (Standing or Sitting)		2.2	2.3	2.5	2.6	2.7	2.8	3.0	3.1	3.2
Driving										
Automobile or light truck		1.8	1.9	2.0	2.1	2.2	2.3	2.4	2.5	2.6
Changing oil		2.4	2.5	2.7	2.8	3.0	3.1	3.3	3.4	3.6
Drag racing, pushing a car		5.3	5.6	5.9	6.2	6.5	6.8	7.1	7.5	7.8
Fidgeting (squeezing piece of rubber or hand grip with free hand)		1.3	1.4	1.5	1.5	1.6	1.7	1.8	1.8	1.9
Fidgeting (squirming while stopped for light or traffic)		1.8	1.9	2.0	2.1	2.2	2.3	2.4	2.6	2.7
Heavy truck (semi), tractor, bus		2.6	2.8	2.9	3.1	3.3	3.4	3.6	3.7	3.9
Stopping for 1 min. brisk walk along flat highway during long drives		3.5	3.7	3.9	4.1	4.3	4.6	4.8	5.0	5.2
Tractor-trailer truck driving, long distance		1.5	1.6	1.7	1.8	1.8	1.9	2.0	2.1	2.2
Truck driving, loading and unloading (standing)		5.7	6.0	6.4	6.7	7.1	7.4	7.7	8.1	8.4
Using self-service gas pumps		2.1	2.2	2.4	2.5	2.6	2.7	2.9	3.0	3.1

Calories Expended by Body Weight

Your Body Weight

| 77 | 80 | 83 | 86 | 89 | 92 | 95 | 98 | 101 | 104 | 107 | 110 | 113 | 116 | 119 |
170	176	183	190	196	203	209	216	223	229	236	243	249	256	262
10.9	11.3	11.8	12.2	12.6	13.0	13.4	13.9	14.3	14.7	15.1	15.6	16.0	16.4	16.8
11.4	11.8	12.3	12.7	13.2	13.6	14.1	14.5	15.0	15.4	15.8	16.3	16.7	17.2	17.6
8.2	8.5	8.8	9.1	9.4	9.8	10.1	10.4	10.7	11.0	11.3	11.7	12.0	12.3	12.6
8.1	8.4	8.7	9.0	9.3	9.7	10.0	10.3	10.6	10.9	11.2	11.6	11.9	12.2	12.5
6.5	6.7	7.0	7.2	7.5	7.7	8.0	8.2	8.5	8.7	9.0	9.2	9.5	9.7	10.0
3.4	3.5	3.6	3.8	3.9	4.0	4.2	4.3	4.4	4.6	4.7	4.8	4.9	5.1	5.2
6.7	7.0	7.3	7.5	7.8	8.1	8.3	8.6	8.8	9.1	9.4	9.6	9.9	10.2	10.4
6.7	7.0	7.3	7.5	7.8	8.1	8.3	8.6	8.8	9.1	9.4	9.6	9.9	10.2	10.4
5.4	5.6	5.8	6.0	6.2	6.4	6.7	6.9	7.1	7.3	7.5	7.7	7.9	8.1	8.3
4.0	4.2	4.4	4.5	4.7	4.8	5.0	5.1	5.3	5.5	5.6	5.8	5.9	6.1	6.2
3.4	3.5	3.6	3.8	3.9	4.0	4.2	4.3	4.4	4.6	4.7	4.8	4.9	5.1	5.2
2.7	2.8	2.9	3.0	3.1	3.2	3.3	3.4	3.5	3.6	3.7	3.9	4.0	4.1	4.2
3.7	3.8	4.0	4.1	4.3	4.4	4.6	4.7	4.8	5.0	5.1	5.3	5.4	5.6	5.7
8.1	8.4	8.7	9.0	9.3	9.7	10.0	10.3	10.6	10.9	11.2	11.6	11.9	12.2	12.5
2.0	2.1	2.2	2.2	2.3	2.4	2.5	2.5	2.6	2.7	2.8	2.9	2.9	3.0	3.1
2.8	2.9	3.0	3.1	3.2	3.3	3.4	3.5	3.6	3.7	3.9	4.0	4.1	4.2	4.3
4.0	4.2	4.4	4.5	4.7	4.8	5.0	5.1	5.3	5.5	5.6	5.8	5.9	6.1	6.2
5.4	5.6	5.8	6.0	6.2	6.4	6.7	6.9	7.1	7.3	7.5	7.7	7.9	8.1	8.3
2.3	2.4	2.5	2.6	2.6	2.7	2.8	2.9	3.0	3.1	3.2	3.3	3.4	3.5	3.5
8.8	9.1	9.4	9.8	10.1	10.5	10.8	11.1	11.5	11.8	12.2	12.5	12.9	13.2	13.5
3.2	3.4	3.5	3.6	3.7	3.9	4.0	4.1	4.2	4.4	4.5	4.6	4.7	4.9	5.0

Calories Expended by Body Weight

		Your Body Weight								
	kg	50	53	56	59	62	65	68	71	74
Activity	lb	110	117	123	130	137	143	150	157	163
Drum Playing		3.5	3.7	3.9	4.1	4.3	4.6	4.8	5.0	5.2
Eating										
Sitting		1.3	1.4	1.5	1.5	1.6	1.7	1.8	1.9	1.9
Standing while talking		1.8	1.9	2.0	2.1	2.2	2.3	2.4	2.5	2.6
Electrical Work										
Strenuous		3.1	3.2	3.4	3.6	3.8	4.0	4.2	4.3	4.5
Wiring, inside		2.6	2.8	2.9	3.1	3.3	3.4	3.6	3.7	3.9
Equestrian										
Horse grooming		5.3	5.6	5.9	6.2	6.5	6.8	7.1	7.5	7.8
Horse racing, galloping		7.0	7.4	7.8	8.3	8.7	9.1	9.5	9.9	10.4
Horse racing, trotting		5.7	6.0	6.4	6.7	7.1	7.4	7.7	8.1	8.4
Horse racing, walking		2.3	2.4	2.5	2.7	2.8	3.0	3.1	3.2	3.4
Horseback riding, general		3.5	3.7	3.9	4.1	4.3	4.6	4.8	5.0	5.2
Horseback riding, saddling horse		3.1	3.2	3.4	3.6	3.8	4.0	4.2	4.3	4.5
Horseback riding, trotting		5.7	6.0	6.4	6.7	7.1	7.4	7.7	8.1	8.4
Horseback riding, walking		2.2	2.3	2.5	2.6	2.7	2.8	3.0	3.1	3.2
Farming										
Baling hay, cleaning barn and stalls, poultry work		7.0	7.4	7.8	8.3	8.7	9.1	9.5	9.9	10.4
Chasing cattle, nonstrenuous		3.1	3.2	3.4	3.6	3.8	4.0	4.2	4.3	4.5
Driving harvester or tractor		2.2	2.3	2.5	2.6	2.7	2.8	3.0	3.1	3.2
Feeding cattle		3.9	4.2	4.4	4.6	4.9	5.1	5.4	5.6	5.8
Feeding small animals		3.5	3.7	3.9	4.1	4.3	4.6	4.8	5.0	5.2
Forking straw bales		7.0	7.4	7.8	8.3	8.7	9.1	9.5	9.9	10.4
Grove work (apples, oranges, peaches, pears)		3.9	4.2	4.4	4.6	4.9	5.1	5.4	5.6	5.8
Milking by hand		2.6	2.8	2.9	3.1	3.3	3.4	3.6	3.7	3.9
Milking by machine		1.3	1.4	1.5	1.5	1.6	1.7	1.8	1.9	1.9
Shoveling grain		4.8	5.1	5.4	5.7	6.0	6.3	6.5	6.8	7.1
Fencing		5.3	5.6	5.9	6.2	6.5	6.8	7.1	7.5	7.8
Field Hockey										
Field game (competition, structured)		7.0	7.4	7.8	8.3	8.7	9.1	9.5	9.9	10.4
Practice		6.1	6.5	6.9	7.2	7.6	8.0	8.3	8.7	9.1

Calories Expended by Body Weight

Your Body Weight

77 170	80 176	83 183	86 190	89 196	92 203	95 209	98 216	101 223	104 229	107 236	110 243	113 249	116 256	119 262
5.4	5.6	5.8	6.0	6.2	6.4	6.7	6.9	7.1	7.3	7.5	7.7	7.9	8.1	8.3
2.0	2.1	2.2	2.3	2.3	2.4	2.5	2.6	2.7	2.7	2.8	2.9	3.0	3.0	3.1
2.7	2.8	2.9	3.0	3.1	3.2	3.3	3.4	3.5	3.6	3.7	3.9	4.0	4.1	4.2
4.7	4.9	5.1	5.3	5.5	5.6	5.8	6.0	6.2	6.4	6.6	6.7	6.9	7.1	7.3
4.0	4.2	4.4	4.5	4.7	4.8	5.0	5.1	5.3	5.5	5.6	5.8	5.9	6.1	6.2
8.1	8.4	8.7	9.0	9.3	9.7	10.0	10.3	10.6	10.9	11.2	11.6	11.9	12.2	12.5
10.8	11.2	11.6	12.0	12.5	12.9	13.3	13.7	14.1	14.6	15.0	15.4	15.8	16.2	16.7
8.8	9.1	9.4	9.8	10.1	10.5	10.8	11.1	11.5	11.8	12.2	12.5	12.9	13.2	13.5
3.5	3.6	3.8	3.9	4.0	4.2	4.3	4.5	4.6	4.7	4.9	5.0	5.1	5.3	5.4
5.4	5.6	5.8	6.0	6.2	6.4	6.7	6.9	7.1	7.3	7.5	7.7	7.9	8.1	8.3
4.7	4.9	5.1	5.3	5.5	5.6	5.8	6.0	6.2	6.4	6.6	6.7	6.9	7.1	7.3
8.8	9.1	9.4	9.8	10.1	10.5	10.8	11.1	11.5	11.8	12.2	12.5	12.9	13.2	13.5
3.4	3.5	3.6	3.8	3.9	4.0	4.2	4.3	4.4	4.6	4.7	4.8	4.9	5.1	5.2
10.8	11.2	11.6	12.0	12.5	12.9	13.3	13.7	14.1	14.6	15.0	15.4	15.8	16.2	16.7
4.7	4.9	5.1	5.3	5.5	5.6	5.8	6.0	6.2	6.4	6.6	6.7	6.9	7.1	7.3
3.4	3.5	3.6	3.8	3.9	4.0	4.2	4.3	4.4	4.6	4.7	4.8	4.9	5.1	5.2
6.1	6.3	6.5	6.8	7.0	7.2	7.5	7.7	8.0	8.2	8.4	8.7	8.9	9.1	9.4
5.4	5.6	5.8	6.0	6.2	6.4	6.7	6.9	7.1	7.3	7.5	7.7	7.9	8.1	8.3
10.8	11.2	11.6	12.0	12.5	12.9	13.3	13.7	14.1	14.6	15.0	15.4	15.8	16.2	16.7
6.1	6.3	6.5	6.8	7.0	7.2	7.5	7.7	8.0	8.2	8.4	8.7	8.9	9.1	9.4
4.0	4.2	4.4	4.5	4.7	4.8	5.0	5.1	5.3	5.5	5.6	5.8	5.9	6.1	6.2
2.0	2.1	2.2	2.3	2.3	2.4	2.5	2.6	2.7	2.7	2.8	2.9	3.0	3.0	3.1
7.4	7.7	8.0	8.3	8.6	8.9	9.1	9.4	9.7	10.0	10.3	10.6	10.9	11.2	11.5
8.1	8.4	8.7	9.0	9.3	9.7	10.0	10.3	10.6	10.9	11.2	11.6	11.9	12.2	12.5
10.8	11.2	11.6	12.0	12.5	12.9	13.3	13.7	14.1	14.6	15.0	15.4	15.8	16.2	16.7
9.4	9.8	10.2	10.5	10.9	11.3	11.6	12.0	12.4	12.7	13.1	13.5	13.8	14.2	14.6

Calories Expended by Body Weight

					Your Body Weight				
	kg 50	**53**	**56**	**59**	**62**	**65**	**68**	**71**	**74**
Activity	**lb 110**	**117**	**123**	**130**	**137**	**143**	**150**	**157**	**163**
Firefighting									
Climbing ladder with full gear	9.6	10.2	10.8	11.4	11.9	12.5	13.1	13.7	14.2
Forest service, hauling hoses on ground	6.6	7.0	7.4	7.8	8.2	8.6	9.0	9.4	9.8
Forest service, hiking in mountainous terrain	5.3	5.6	5.9	6.2	6.5	6.8	7.1	7.5	7.8
Forest service, working with a Pulaski	5.6	5.9	6.2	6.6	6.9	7.2	7.6	7.9	8.2
Forest service, working with a shovel	5.7	6.1	6.4	6.8	7.1	7.4	7.8	8.1	8.5
General	5.6	6.0	6.3	6.6	7.0	7.3	7.7	8.0	8.3
Fishing									
Boat, sitting	2.2	2.3	2.5	2.6	2.7	2.8	3.0	3.1	3.2
General	3.5	3.7	3.9	4.1	4.3	4.6	4.8	5.0	5.2
Ice, sitting	1.8	1.9	2.0	2.1	2.2	2.3	2.4	2.5	2.6
Riverbank, walking	4.4	4.6	4.9	5.2	5.4	5.7	6.0	6.2	6.5
Riverbank, standing	3.1	3.2	3.4	3.6	3.8	4.0	4.2	4.3	4.5
Stream, in waders	5.3	5.6	5.9	6.2	6.5	6.8	7.1	7.5	7.8
Flute Playing (Sitting)	1.8	1.9	2.0	2.1	2.2	2.3	2.4	2.5	2.6
Flying Airplane (Pilot, Copilot, Navigator)	1.8	1.9	2.0	2.1	2.2	2.3	2.4	2.5	2.6
Football									
Competition (structured play)	7.9	8.3	8.8	9.3	9.8	10.2	10.7	11.2	11.7
Playing catch	2.2	2.3	2.5	2.6	2.7	2.8	3.0	3.1	3.2
Touch, flag, general	7.0	7.4	7.8	8.3	8.7	9.1	9.5	9.9	10.4
Forestry									
Ax, chopping fast	14.9	15.8	16.7	17.6	18.4	19.3	20.2	21.1	22.0
Ax, chopping slow	4.4	4.6	4.9	5.2	5.4	5.7	6.0	6.2	6.5
Barking trees	6.1	6.5	6.9	7.2	7.6	8.0	8.3	8.7	9.1
Carrying logs	9.6	10.2	10.8	11.4	11.9	12.5	13.1	13.7	14.2
Felling trees	7.0	7.4	7.8	8.3	8.7	9.1	9.5	9.9	10.4
General	7.0	7.4	7.8	8.3	8.7	9.1	9.5	9.9	10.4
Hoeing	4.4	4.6	4.9	5.2	5.4	5.7	6.0	6.2	6.5
Planting by hand	5.3	5.6	5.9	6.2	6.5	6.8	7.1	7.5	7.8

Calories Expended by Body Weight

Your Body Weight

77 170	80 176	83 183	86 190	89 196	92 203	95 209	98 216	101 223	104 229	107 236	110 243	113 249	116 256	119 262
14.8	15.4	16.0	16.6	17.1	17.7	18.3	18.9	19.4	20.0	20.6	21.2	21.8	22.3	22.9
10.2	10.6	11.0	11.4	11.8	12.2	12.6	12.9	13.3	13.7	14.1	14.5	14.9	15.3	15.7
8.1	8.4	8.7	9.0	9.3	9.7	10.0	10.3	10.6	10.9	11.2	11.6	11.9	12.2	12.5
8.6	8.9	9.3	9.6	9.9	10.3	10.6	10.9	11.3	11.6	11.9	12.3	12.6	12.9	13.3
8.8	9.2	9.5	9.8	10.2	10.5	10.9	11.2	11.6	11.9	12.2	12.6	12.9	13.3	13.6
8.7	9.0	9.3	9.7	10.0	10.4	10.7	11.0	11.4	11.7	12.0	12.4	12.7	13.1	13.4
3.4	3.5	3.6	3.8	3.9	4.0	4.2	4.3	4.4	4.6	4.7	4.8	4.9	5.1	5.2
5.4	5.6	5.8	6.0	6.2	6.4	6.7	6.9	7.1	7.3	7.5	7.7	7.9	8.1	8.3
2.7	2.8	2.9	3.0	3.1	3.2	3.3	3.4	3.5	3.6	3.7	3.9	4.0	4.1	4.2
6.7	7.0	7.3	7.5	7.8	8.1	8.3	8.6	8.8	9.1	9.4	9.6	9.9	10.2	10.4
4.7	4.9	5.1	5.3	5.5	5.6	5.8	6.0	6.2	6.4	6.6	6.7	6.9	7.1	7.3
8.1	8.4	8.7	9.0	9.3	9.7	10.0	10.3	10.6	10.9	11.2	11.6	11.9	12.2	12.5
2.7	2.8	2.9	3.0	3.1	3.2	3.3	3.4	3.5	3.6	3.7	3.9	4.0	4.1	4.2
2.7	2.8	2.9	3.0	3.1	3.2	3.3	3.4	3.5	3.6	3.7	3.9	4.0	4.1	4.2
12.1	12.6	13.1	13.5	14.0	14.5	15.0	15.4	15.9	16.4	16.9	17.3	17.8	18.3	18.7
3.4	3.5	3.6	3.8	3.9	4.0	4.2	4.3	4.4	4.6	4.7	4.8	4.9	5.1	5.2
10.8	11.2	11.6	12.0	12.5	12.9	13.3	13.7	14.1	14.6	15.0	15.4	15.8	16.2	16.7
22.9	23.8	24.7	25.6	26.5	27.4	28.3	29.2	30.0	30.9	31.8	32.7	33.6	34.5	35.4
6.7	7.0	7.3	7.5	7.8	8.1	8.3	8.6	8.8	9.1	9.4	9.6	9.9	10.2	10.4
9.4	9.8	10.2	10.5	10.9	11.3	11.6	12.0	12.4	12.7	13.1	13.5	13.8	14.2	14.6
14.8	15.4	16.0	16.6	17.1	17.7	18.3	18.9	19.4	20.0	20.6	21.2	21.8	22.3	22.9
10.8	11.2	11.6	12.0	12.5	12.9	13.3	13.7	14.1	14.6	15.0	15.4	15.8	16.2	16.7
10.8	11.2	11.6	12.0	12.5	12.9	13.3	13.7	14.1	14.6	15.0	15.4	15.8	16.2	16.7
6.7	7.0	7.3	7.5	7.8	8.1	8.3	8.6	8.8	9.1	9.4	9.6	9.9	10.2	10.4
8.1	8.4	8.7	9.0	9.3	9.7	10.0	10.3	10.6	10.9	11.2	11.6	11.9	12.2	12.5

	Calories Expended by Body Weight								
	Your Body Weight								
Activity	**kg 50 / lb 110**	**53 / 117**	**56 / 123**	**59 / 130**	**62 / 137**	**65 / 143**	**68 / 150**	**71 / 157**	**74 / 163**
Forestry (cont.)									
Sawing by hand	6.1	6.5	6.9	7.2	7.6	8.0	8.3	8.7	9.1
Sawing, power tools	3.9	4.2	4.4	4.6	4.9	5.1	5.4	5.6	5.8
Trimming trees	7.9	8.3	8.8	9.3	9.8	10.2	10.7	11.2	11.7
Weeding	3.5	3.7	3.9	4.1	4.3	4.6	4.8	5.0	5.2
Frisbee									
General	2.6	2.8	2.9	3.1	3.3	3.4	3.6	3.7	3.9
Ultimate Frisbee (competition)	5.4	5.8	6.1	6.4	6.7	7.1	7.4	7.7	8.0
Gardening									
Applying fertilizer, lime, seeding a lawn	2.2	2.3	2.5	2.6	2.7	2.8	3.0	3.1	3.2
Broom sweeping decks	2.6	2.8	2.9	3.1	3.2	3.4	3.5	3.7	3.8
Cutting lawn (manual mower)	5.3	5.6	5.9	6.3	6.6	6.9	7.2	7.5	7.8
Cutting lawn (push power mower)	3.9	4.2	4.4	4.6	4.9	5.1	5.4	5.6	5.8
Cutting lawn (riding mower)	2.2	2.3	2.5	2.6	2.7	2.8	3.0	3.1	3.2
Picking up in yard, light effort	2.6	2.8	2.9	3.1	3.3	3.4	3.6	3.7	3.9
Planting seedlings, shrubs, bushes, flowers, bulbs	3.5	3.7	3.9	4.1	4.3	4.6	4.8	5.0	5.2
Planting trees	3.9	4.2	4.4	4.6	4.9	5.1	5.4	5.6	5.8
Raking leaves	3.5	3.7	3.9	4.1	4.3	4.6	4.8	5.0	5.2
Sacking grass, leaves	3.5	3.7	3.9	4.1	4.3	4.6	4.8	5.0	5.2
Tilling garden (heavy power tools)	5.3	5.6	5.9	6.2	6.5	6.8	7.1	7.5	7.8
Trimming shrubs or trees, manual cutter	3.9	4.2	4.4	4.6	4.9	5.1	5.4	5.6	5.8
Trimming shrubs or trees, power cutter	3.1	3.2	3.4	3.6	3.8	4.0	4.2	4.3	4.5
Watering lawn or garden, standing or walking	1.3	1.4	1.5	1.5	1.6	1.7	1.8	1.9	1.9
Weeding, cultivating garden	3.9	4.2	4.4	4.6	4.9	5.1	5.4	5.6	5.8
Golf									
Carrying clubs (caddy)	4.8	5.1	5.4	5.7	6.0	6.3	6.5	6.8	7.1
Driving range	2.6	2.8	2.9	3.1	3.3	3.4	3.6	3.7	3.9
General	3.9	4.2	4.4	4.6	4.9	5.1	5.4	5.6	5.8
Pulling clubs in cart	4.4	4.6	4.9	5.2	5.4	5.7	6.0	6.2	6.5
Using power cart	3.1	3.2	3.4	3.6	3.8	4.0	4.2	4.3	4.5

Calories Expended by Body Weight

Your Body Weight

77 170	80 176	83 183	86 190	89 196	92 203	95 209	98 216	101 223	104 229	107 236	110 243	113 249	116 256	119 262
9.4	9.8	10.2	10.5	10.9	11.3	11.6	12.0	12.4	12.7	13.1	13.5	13.8	14.2	14.6
6.1	6.3	6.5	6.8	7.0	7.2	7.5	7.7	8.0	8.2	8.4	8.7	8.9	9.1	9.4
12.1	12.6	13.1	13.5	14.0	14.5	15.0	15.4	15.9	16.4	16.9	17.3	17.8	18.3	18.7
5.4	5.6	5.8	6.0	6.2	6.4	6.7	6.9	7.1	7.3	7.5	7.7	7.9	8.1	8.3
4.0	4.2	4.4	4.5	4.7	4.8	5.0	5.1	5.3	5.5	5.6	5.8	5.9	6.1	6.2
8.4	8.7	9.0	9.3	9.7	10.0	10.3	10.6	11.0	11.3	11.6	11.9	12.3	12.6	12.9
3.4	3.5	3.6	3.8	3.9	4.0	4.2	4.3	4.4	4.6	4.7	4.8	4.9	5.1	5.2
4.0	4.2	4.3	4.5	4.6	4.8	4.9	5.1	5.3	5.4	5.6	5.7	5.9	6.0	6.2
8.2	8.5	8.8	9.1	9.4	9.8	10.1	10.4	10.7	11.0	11.3	11.7	12.0	12.3	12.6
6.1	6.3	6.5	6.8	7.0	7.2	7.5	7.7	8.0	8.2	8.4	8.7	8.9	9.1	9.4
3.4	3.5	3.6	3.8	3.9	4.0	4.2	4.3	4.4	4.6	4.7	4.8	4.9	5.1	5.2
4.0	4.2	4.4	4.5	4.7	4.8	5.0	5.1	5.3	5.5	5.6	5.8	5.9	6.1	6.2
5.4	5.6	5.8	6.0	6.2	6.4	6.7	6.9	7.1	7.3	7.5	7.7	7.9	8.1	8.3
6.1	6.3	6.5	6.8	7.0	7.2	7.5	7.7	8.0	8.2	8.4	8.7	8.9	9.1	9.4
5.4	5.6	5.8	6.0	6.2	6.4	6.7	6.9	7.1	7.3	7.5	7.7	7.9	8.1	8.3
5.4	5.6	5.8	6.0	6.2	6.4	6.7	6.9	7.1	7.3	7.5	7.7	7.9	8.1	8.3
8.1	8.4	8.7	9.0	9.3	9.7	10.0	10.3	10.6	10.9	11.2	11.6	11.9	12.2	12.5
6.1	6.3	6.5	6.8	7.0	7.2	7.5	7.7	8.0	8.2	8.4	8.7	8.9	9.1	9.4
4.7	4.9	5.1	5.3	5.5	5.6	5.8	6.0	6.2	6.4	6.6	6.7	6.9	7.1	7.3
2.0	2.1	2.2	2.3	2.3	2.4	2.5	2.6	2.7	2.7	2.8	2.9	3.0	3.0	3.1
6.1	6.3	6.5	6.8	7.0	7.2	7.5	7.7	8.0	8.2	8.4	8.7	8.9	9.1	9.4
7.4	7.7	8.0	8.3	8.6	8.9	9.1	9.4	9.7	10.0	10.3	10.6	10.9	11.2	11.5
4.0	4.2	4.4	4.5	4.7	4.8	5.0	5.1	5.3	5.5	5.6	5.8	5.9	6.1	6.2
6.1	6.3	6.5	6.8	7.0	7.2	7.5	7.7	8.0	8.2	8.4	8.7	8.9	9.1	9.4
6.7	7.0	7.3	7.5	7.8	8.1	8.3	8.6	8.8	9.1	9.4	9.6	9.9	10.2	10.4
4.7	4.9	5.1	5.3	5.5	5.6	5.8	6.0	6.2	6.4	6.6	6.7	6.9	7.1	7.3

Calories Expended by Body Weight

Activity	kg 50 lb 110	53 117	56 123	59 130	62 137	65 143	68 150	71 157	74 163
Golf—Miniature	2.6	2.8	2.9	3.1	3.3	3.4	3.6	3.7	3.9
Grocery Shopping (with Cart)	3.1	3.2	3.4	3.6	3.8	4.0	4.2	4.3	4.5
Guitar Playing									
Classical, folk (sitting)	1.8	1.9	2.0	2.1	2.2	2.3	2.4	2.5	2.6
Rock 'n' roll band (standing)	2.6	2.8	2.9	3.1	3.3	3.4	3.6	3.7	3.9
Gymnastics (General)	3.5	3.7	3.9	4.1	4.3	4.6	4.8	5.0	5.2
Hacky Sack	3.5	3.7	3.9	4.1	4.3	4.6	4.8	5.0	5.2
Handball									
General	10.5	11.1	11.8	12.4	13.0	13.7	14.3	14.9	15.5
Team	7.0	7.4	7.8	8.3	8.7	9.1	9.5	9.9	10.4
Hang Gliding	3.1	3.2	3.4	3.6	3.8	4.0	4.2	4.3	4.5
Hanging Storm Windows	4.4	4.6	4.9	5.2	5.4	5.7	6.0	6.2	6.5
Health Club Exercise (General, Unstructured)	4.8	5.1	5.4	5.7	6.0	6.3	6.5	6.8	7.1
Heavy Tools									
Hand tools (shovel, pick bar, spade)	7.0	7.4	7.8	8.3	8.7	9.1	9.5	9.9	10.4
Power tools (pneumatic jackhammers, drills)	5.3	5.6	5.9	6.2	6.5	6.8	7.1	7.5	7.8
Hiking (Hills and Mountains)	5.3	5.6	5.9	6.2	6.5	6.8	7.1	7.5	7.8
Horn Playing	1.8	1.9	2.0	2.1	2.2	2.3	2.4	2.5	2.6
Horseshoe Pitching (Quoits)	2.6	2.8	2.9	3.1	3.3	3.4	3.6	3.7	3.9
Hot Tub (Sitting and Relaxing)	1.0	1.0	1.1	1.1	1.2	1.3	1.3	1.4	1.4
Hunting									
Bow and arrow, crossbow	2.2	2.3	2.5	2.6	2.7	2.8	3.0	3.1	3.2
Deer, elk, large game	5.3	5.6	5.9	6.2	6.5	6.8	7.1	7.5	7.8
Duck, wading	2.2	2.3	2.5	2.6	2.7	2.8	3.0	3.1	3.2
General (small game)	4.4	4.6	4.9	5.2	5.4	5.7	6.0	6.2	6.5

Calories Expended by Body Weight

Your Body Weight

77 170	80 176	83 183	86 190	89 196	92 203	95 209	98 216	101 223	104 229	107 236	110 243	113 249	116 256	119 262
4.0	4.2	4.4	4.5	4.7	4.8	5.0	5.1	5.3	5.5	5.6	5.8	5.9	6.1	6.2
4.7	4.9	5.1	5.3	5.5	5.6	5.8	6.0	6.2	6.4	6.6	6.7	6.9	7.1	7.3
2.7	2.8	2.9	3.0	3.1	3.2	3.3	3.4	3.5	3.6	3.7	3.9	4.0	4.1	4.2
4.0	4.2	4.4	4.5	4.7	4.8	5.0	5.1	5.3	5.5	5.6	5.8	5.9	6.1	6.2
5.4	5.6	5.8	6.0	6.2	6.4	6.7	6.9	7.1	7.3	7.5	7.7	7.9	8.1	8.3
5.4	5.6	5.8	6.0	6.2	6.4	6.7	6.9	7.1	7.3	7.5	7.7	7.9	8.1	8.3
16.2	16.8	17.4	18.1	18.7	19.3	20.0	20.6	21.2	21.8	22.5	23.1	23.7	24.4	25.0
10.8	11.2	11.6	12.0	12.5	12.9	13.3	13.7	14.1	14.6	15.0	15.4	15.8	16.2	16.7
4.7	4.9	5.1	5.3	5.5	5.6	5.8	6.0	6.2	6.4	6.6	6.7	6.9	7.1	7.3
6.7	7.0	7.3	7.5	7.8	8.1	8.3	8.6	8.8	9.1	9.4	9.6	9.9	10.2	10.4
7.4	7.7	8.0	8.3	8.6	8.9	9.1	9.4	9.7	10.0	10.3	10.6	10.9	11.2	11.5
10.8	11.2	11.6	12.0	12.5	12.9	13.3	13.7	14.1	14.6	15.0	15.4	15.8	16.2	16.7
8.1	8.4	8.7	9.0	9.3	9.7	10.0	10.3	10.6	10.9	11.2	11.6	11.9	12.2	12.5
8.1	8.4	8.7	9.0	9.3	9.7	10.0	10.3	10.6	10.9	11.2	11.6	11.9	12.2	12.5
2.7	2.8	2.9	3.0	3.1	3.2	3.3	3.4	3.5	3.6	3.7	3.9	4.0	4.1	4.2
4.0	4.2	4.4	4.5	4.7	4.8	5.0	5.1	5.3	5.5	5.6	5.8	5.9	6.1	6.2
1.5	1.6	1.6	1.7	1.7	1.8	1.8	1.9	2.0	2.0	2.1	2.1	2.2	2.3	2.3
3.4	3.5	3.6	3.8	3.9	4.0	4.2	4.3	4.4	4.6	4.7	4.8	4.9	5.1	5.2
8.1	8.4	8.7	9.0	9.3	9.7	10.0	10.3	10.6	10.9	11.2	11.6	11.9	12.2	12.5
3.4	3.5	3.6	3.8	3.9	4.0	4.2	4.3	4.4	4.6	4.7	4.8	4.9	5.1	5.2
6.7	7.0	7.3	7.5	7.8	8.1	8.3	8.6	8.8	9.1	9.4	9.6	9.9	10.2	10.4

Calories Expended by Body Weight

Your Body Weight

Activity	kg 50 lb 110	53 117	56 123	59 130	62 137	65 143	68 150	71 157	74 163
Hunting (cont.)									
Pheasant or grouse	5.3	5.6	5.9	6.2	6.5	6.8	7.1	7.5	7.8
Pistol shooting or trapshooting, standing	2.2	2.3	2.5	2.6	2.7	2.8	3.0	3.1	3.2
Ice Dancing (Vigorous, Competition)	8.9	9.5	10.0	10.5	11.1	11.6	12.1	12.7	13.2
Ice Hockey									
Game (structured)	7.0	7.4	7.8	8.3	8.7	9.1	9.5	9.9	10.4
Practice	6.6	7.0	7.4	7.7	8.1	8.5	8.9	9.3	9.7
Ice Sailing	3.8	4.0	4.2	4.4	4.7	4.9	5.1	5.3	5.6
Ice-Skating									
Less than 9 mph	4.8	5.1	5.4	5.7	6.0	6.3	6.5	6.8	7.1
More than 9 mph	7.9	8.3	8.8	9.3	9.8	10.2	10.7	11.2	11.7
Competition, speed skating	13.1	13.9	14.7	15.5	16.3	17.1	17.9	18.6	19.4
In-Line Skating									
Casual	6.7	7.0	7.4	7.8	8.2	8.6	9.0	9.4	9.8
Vigorous, 12.4 mph on asphalt	10.6	11.2	11.9	12.5	13.1	13.8	14.4	15.0	15.7
In-Line Skiing									
Double-pole technique, 10.3 mph, highly trained athletes	17.7	18.8	19.9	20.9	22.0	23.1	24.1	25.2	26.3
Double-pole technique, 11.2 mph, highly trained athletes	20.4	21.6	22.8	24.0	25.3	26.5	27.7	28.9	30.1
Skate technique, 9 mph, highly trained athletes	17.4	18.5	19.5	20.6	21.6	22.7	23.7	24.8	25.8
Skate technique, 10.3 mph, highly trained athletes	19.7	20.9	22.1	23.2	24.4	25.6	26.8	28.0	29.1
Skate technique, 11.2 mph, highly trained athletes	22.6	24.0	25.3	26.7	28.1	29.4	30.8	32.1	33.5
Ironing Clothes (Standing)	2.0	2.1	2.3	2.4	2.5	2.6	2.7	2.9	3.0
Jai Alai	10.5	11.1	11.8	12.4	13.0	13.7	14.3	14.9	15.5

Calories Expended by Body Weight

Your Body Weight

77 170	80 176	83 183	86 190	89 196	92 203	95 209	98 216	101 223	104 229	107 236	110 243	113 249	116 256	119 262
8.1	8.4	8.7	9.0	9.3	9.7	10.0	10.3	10.6	10.9	11.2	11.6	11.9	12.2	12.5
3.4	3.5	3.6	3.8	3.9	4.0	4.2	4.3	4.4	4.6	4.7	4.8	4.9	5.1	5.2
13.7	14.3	14.8	15.4	15.9	16.4	17.0	17.5	18.0	18.6	19.1	19.6	20.2	20.7	21.2
10.8	11.2	11.6	12.0	12.5	12.9	13.3	13.7	14.1	14.6	15.0	15.4	15.8	16.2	16.7
10.1	10.5	10.9	11.3	11.7	12.1	12.5	12.9	13.3	13.7	14.0	14.4	14.8	15.2	15.6
5.8	6.0	6.2	6.5	6.7	6.9	7.1	7.4	7.6	7.8	8.1	8.3	8.5	8.7	9.0
7.4	7.7	8.0	8.3	8.6	8.9	9.1	9.4	9.7	10.0	10.3	10.6	10.9	11.2	11.5
12.1	12.6	13.1	13.5	14.0	14.5	15.0	15.4	15.9	16.4	16.9	17.3	17.8	18.3	18.7
20.2	21.0	21.8	22.6	23.4	24.2	24.9	25.7	26.5	27.3	28.1	28.9	29.7	30.5	31.2
10.2	10.6	11.0	11.4	11.8	12.2	12.6	13.0	13.4	13.8	14.2	14.6	15.0	15.4	15.8
16.3	16.9	17.6	18.2	18.8	19.5	20.1	20.8	21.4	22.0	22.7	23.3	23.9	24.6	25.2
27.3	28.4	29.5	30.5	31.6	32.7	33.7	34.8	35.8	36.9	38.0	39.0	40.1	41.2	42.2
31.4	32.6	33.8	35.0	36.3	37.5	38.7	39.9	41.1	42.4	43.6	44.8	46.0	47.3	48.5
26.8	27.9	28.9	30.0	31.0	32.1	33.1	34.2	35.2	36.3	37.3	38.3	39.4	40.4	41.5
30.3	31.5	32.7	33.9	35.0	36.2	37.4	38.6	39.8	41.0	42.1	43.3	44.5	45.7	46.9
34.8	36.2	37.6	38.9	40.3	41.6	43.0	44.3	45.7	47.1	48.4	49.8	51.1	52.5	53.9
3.1	3.2	3.3	3.5	3.6	3.7	3.8	3.9	4.1	4.2	4.3	4.4	4.5	4.7	4.8
16.2	16.8	17.4	18.1	18.7	19.3	20.0	20.6	21.2	21.8	22.5	23.1	23.7	24.4	25.0

Calories Expended by Body Weight

Activity	kg 50 lb 110	53 117	56 123	59 130	62 137	65 143	68 150	71 157	74 163
Jazzercise									
Casual	5.1	5.4	5.7	6.0	6.3	6.6	6.9	7.2	7.5
Extreme	7.1	7.6	8.0	8.4	8.9	9.3	9.7	10.1	10.6
Moderate	5.8	6.1	6.5	6.8	7.2	7.5	7.9	8.2	8.5
JazzerStep, 6–8 in. bench, (120 beats/min.)	7.7	8.1	8.6	9.0	9.5	10.0	10.4	10.9	11.3
Jet Ski—Wave Running	6.1	6.5	6.9	7.2	7.6	8.0	8.3	8.7	9.1
Judo	8.8	9.3	9.8	10.3	10.9	11.4	11.9	12.4	13.0
Juggling	3.5	3.7	3.9	4.1	4.3	4.6	4.8	5.0	5.2
Jujitsu	8.6	9.1	9.6	10.2	10.7	11.2	11.7	12.2	12.7
Jump Rope									
70 turns/min.	8.5	9.0	9.5	10.0	10.5	11.1	11.6	12.1	12.6
80 turns/min.	8.6	9.1	9.6	10.2	10.7	11.2	11.7	12.2	12.7
110 turns /min.	9.3	9.9	10.4	11.0	11.5	12.1	12.6	13.2	13.8
120 turns/min.	9.6	10.2	10.8	11.4	11.9	12.5	13.1	13.7	14.2
125 turns/min., girls 11–13 years old	9.0	9.5	10.1	10.6	11.2	11.7	12.2	12.8	13.3
125 turns/min.	9.9	10.5	11.1	11.6	12.2	12.8	13.4	14.0	14.6
130 turns/min., women	10.3	10.9	11.6	12.2	12.8	13.4	14.0	14.7	15.3
130 turns/min., men	10.6	11.2	11.9	12.5	13.1	13.8	14.4	15.0	15.7
135 turns/min., girls 11–13 years old	9.1	9.7	10.2	10.8	11.3	11.9	12.4	13.0	13.5
135 turns/min., men	10.9	11.5	12.2	12.8	13.5	14.1	14.8	15.4	16.1
145 turns/min., women	10.4	11.0	11.7	12.3	12.9	13.5	14.2	14.8	15.4
145 turns/min., men	10.9	11.6	12.3	12.9	13.6	14.2	14.9	15.5	16.2
Karate Kata									
15 continuous kata, 30 sec. pace	7.8	8.2	8.7	9.2	9.6	10.1	10.6	11.0	11.5
15 kata intermittently, 1 min. rest between kata	4.3	4.6	4.8	5.1	5.4	5.6	5.9	6.1	6.4
Kayaking									
No wash-riding technique, elite athletes	11.4	12.1	12.7	13.4	14.1	14.8	15.5	16.2	16.8

Calories Expended by Body Weight

						Your Body Weight								
77	**80**	**83**	**86**	**89**	**92**	**95**	**98**	**101**	**104**	**107**	**110**	**113**	**116**	**119**
170	**176**	**183**	**190**	**196**	**203**	**209**	**216**	**223**	**229**	**236**	**243**	**249**	**256**	**262**

7.8	8.1	8.5	8.8	9.1	9.4	9.7	10.0	10.3	10.6	10.9	11.2	11.5	11.8	12.1
11.0	11.4	11.9	12.3	12.7	13.1	13.6	14.0	14.4	14.9	15.3	15.7	16.1	16.6	17.0
8.9	9.2	9.6	9.9	10.3	10.6	11.0	11.3	11.7	12.0	12.4	12.7	13.1	13.4	13.7
11.8	12.3	12.7	13.2	13.6	14.1	14.6	15.0	15.5	15.9	16.4	16.9	17.3	17.8	18.2

9.4	9.8	10.2	10.5	10.9	11.3	11.6	12.0	12.4	12.7	13.1	13.5	13.8	14.2	14.6

13.5	14.0	14.5	15.1	15.6	16.1	16.6	17.2	17.7	18.2	18.7	19.3	19.8	20.3	20.8

5.4	5.6	5.8	6.0	6.2	6.4	6.7	6.9	7.1	7.3	7.5	7.7	7.9	8.1	8.3

13.3	13.8	14.3	14.8	15.3	15.8	16.4	16.9	17.4	17.9	18.4	18.9	19.5	20.0	20.5

13.1	13.6	14.1	14.6	15.1	15.6	16.2	16.7	17.2	17.7	18.2	18.7	19.2	19.7	20.2
13.3	13.8	14.3	14.8	15.3	15.8	16.4	16.9	17.4	17.9	18.4	18.9	19.5	20.0	20.5
14.3	14.9	15.4	16.0	16.5	17.1	17.7	18.2	18.8	19.3	19.9	20.4	21.0	21.6	22.1
14.8	15.4	16.0	16.6	17.1	17.7	18.3	18.9	19.4	20.0	20.6	21.2	21.8	22.3	22.9
13.9	14.4	14.9	15.5	16.0	16.6	17.1	17.6	18.2	18.7	19.2	19.8	20.3	20.9	21.4

15.2	15.8	16.4	17.0	17.6	18.2	18.8	19.3	19.9	20.5	21.1	21.7	22.3	22.9	23.5
15.9	16.5	17.1	17.8	18.4	19.0	19.6	20.2	20.9	21.5	22.1	22.7	23.3	24.0	24.6
16.3	16.9	17.6	18.2	18.8	19.5	20.1	20.8	21.4	22.0	22.7	23.3	23.9	24.6	25.2
14.1	14.6	15.2	15.7	16.3	16.8	17.4	17.9	18.5	19.0	19.6	20.1	20.7	21.2	21.8

16.7	17.4	18.0	18.7	19.3	20.0	20.6	21.3	21.9	22.6	23.2	23.9	24.5	25.2	25.8
16.0	16.7	17.3	17.9	18.5	19.2	19.8	20.4	21.0	21.7	22.3	22.9	23.5	24.2	24.8
16.8	17.5	18.2	18.8	19.5	20.1	20.8	21.4	22.1	22.8	23.4	24.1	24.7	25.4	26.0

12.0	12.4	12.9	13.4	13.8	14.3	14.8	15.2	15.7	16.2	16.6	17.1	17.6	18.0	18.5
6.7	6.9	7.2	7.4	7.7	8.0	8.2	8.5	8.7	9.0	9.3	9.5	9.8	10.0	10.3

17.5	18.2	18.9	19.6	20.2	20.9	21.6	22.3	23.0	23.7	24.3	25.0	25.7	26.4	27.1

Calories Expended by Body Weight

		Your Body Weight								
Activity	**kg** **lb**	**50** **110**	**53** **117**	**56** **123**	**59** **130**	**62** **137**	**65** **143**	**68** **150**	**71** **157**	**74** **163**
Kayaking (cont.)										
Recreational		4.6	4.8	5.1	5.4	5.6	5.9	6.2	6.5	6.7
Wash-riding technique, elite athletes		10.1	10.7	11.3	11.9	12.5	13.1	13.7	14.3	14.9
Kick Boxing		8.8	9.4	9.9	10.4	11.0	11.5	12.0	12.5	13.1
Kickball		6.1	6.5	6.9	7.2	7.6	8.0	8.3	8.7	9.1
Lacrosse										
Game (competition, structured)		7.3	7.7	8.2	8.6	9.0	9.5	9.9	10.3	10.8
Practice		6.1	6.5	6.9	7.2	7.6	8.0	8.3	8.7	9.1
Laying Materials										
Carpet		3.9	4.2	4.4	4.6	4.9	5.1	5.4	5.6	5.8
Crushed rock		4.4	4.6	4.9	5.2	5.4	5.7	6.0	6.2	6.5
Sod		4.4	4.6	4.9	5.2	5.4	5.7	6.0	6.2	6.5
Tile or linoleum		3.9	4.2	4.4	4.6	4.9	5.1	5.4	5.6	5.8
Locksmith		3.1	3.2	3.4	3.6	3.8	4.0	4.2	4.3	4.5
Luge		6.5	6.9	7.3	7.7	8.1	8.5	8.9	9.3	9.7
Machine Tooling										
Machining, working sheet metal		2.2	2.3	2.5	2.6	2.7	2.8	3.0	3.1	3.2
Operating lathe		2.6	2.8	2.9	3.1	3.3	3.4	3.6	3.7	3.9
Operating punch press		4.4	4.6	4.9	5.2	5.4	5.7	6.0	6.2	6.5
Tapping and drilling		3.5	3.7	3.9	4.1	4.3	4.6	4.8	5.0	5.2
Welding		2.6	2.8	2.9	3.1	3.3	3.4	3.6	3.7	3.9
Making Bed		1.8	1.9	2.0	2.1	2.2	2.3	2.4	2.5	2.6
Maple Syruping—Sugar Bushing		4.4	4.6	4.9	5.2	5.4	5.7	6.0	6.2	6.5
Marching (Rapidly, Military Style, Cadence)		5.7	6.0	6.4	6.7	7.1	7.4	7.7	8.1	8.4
Marching Band										
Drum major (walking)		3.1	3.2	3.4	3.6	3.8	4.0	4.2	4.3	4.5
Playing instrument, baton twirling (walking)		3.5	3.7	3.9	4.1	4.3	4.6	4.8	5.0	5.2

Calories Expended by Body Weight

					Your Body Weight									
77	**80**	**83**	**86**	**89**	**92**	**95**	**98**	**101**	**104**	**107**	**110**	**113**	**116**	**119**
170	**176**	**183**	**190**	**196**	**203**	**209**	**216**	**223**	**229**	**236**	**243**	**249**	**256**	**262**
7.0	7.3	7.6	7.8	8.1	8.4	8.6	8.9	9.2	9.5	9.7	10.0	10.3	10.6	10.8
15.5	16.1	16.7	17.3	17.9	18.5	19.1	19.7	20.3	20.9	21.5	22.1	22.7	23.3	23.9
13.6	14.1	14.7	15.2	15.7	16.3	16.8	17.3	17.9	18.4	18.9	19.4	20.0	20.5	21.0
9.4	9.8	10.2	10.5	10.9	11.3	11.6	12.0	12.4	12.7	13.1	13.5	13.8	14.2	14.6
11.2	11.6	12.1	12.5	13.0	13.4	13.8	14.3	14.7	15.1	15.6	16.0	16.5	16.9	17.3
9.4	9.8	10.2	10.5	10.9	11.3	11.6	12.0	12.4	12.7	13.1	13.5	13.8	14.2	14.6
6.1	6.3	6.5	6.8	7.0	7.2	7.5	7.7	8.0	8.2	8.4	8.7	8.9	9.1	9.4
6.7	7.0	7.3	7.5	7.8	8.1	8.3	8.6	8.8	9.1	9.4	9.6	9.9	10.2	10.4
6.7	7.0	7.3	7.5	7.8	8.1	8.3	8.6	8.8	9.1	9.4	9.6	9.9	10.2	10.4
6.1	6.3	6.5	6.8	7.0	7.2	7.5	7.7	8.0	8.2	8.4	8.7	8.9	9.1	9.4
4.7	4.9	5.1	5.3	5.5	5.6	5.8	6.0	6.2	6.4	6.6	6.7	6.9	7.1	7.3
10.1	10.5	10.9	11.3	11.7	12.0	12.4	12.8	13.2	13.6	14.0	14.4	14.8	15.2	15.6
3.4	3.5	3.6	3.8	3.9	4.0	4.2	4.3	4.4	4.6	4.7	4.8	4.9	5.1	5.2
4.0	4.2	4.4	4.5	4.7	4.8	5.0	5.1	5.3	5.5	5.6	5.8	5.9	6.1	6.2
6.7	7.0	7.3	7.5	7.8	8.1	8.3	8.6	8.8	9.1	9.4	9.6	9.9	10.2	10.4
5.4	5.6	5.8	6.0	6.2	6.4	6.7	6.9	7.1	7.3	7.5	7.7	7.9	8.1	8.3
4.0	4.2	4.4	4.5	4.7	4.8	5.0	5.1	5.3	5.5	5.6	5.8	5.9	6.1	6.2
2.7	2.8	2.9	3.0	3.1	3.2	3.3	3.4	3.5	3.6	3.7	3.9	4.0	4.1	4.2
6.7	7.0	7.3	7.5	7.8	8.1	8.3	8.6	8.8	9.1	9.4	9.6	9.9	10.2	10.4
8.8	9.1	9.4	9.8	10.1	10.5	10.8	11.1	11.5	11.8	12.2	12.5	12.9	13.2	13.5
4.7	4.9	5.1	5.3	5.5	5.6	5.8	6.0	6.2	6.4	6.6	6.7	6.9	7.1	7.3
5.4	5.6	5.8	6.0	6.2	6.4	6.7	6.9	7.1	7.3	7.5	7.7	7.9	8.1	8.3

Calories Expended by Body Weight

Activity	kg lb	50 110	53 117	56 123	59 130	62 137	65 143	68 150	71 157	74 163
Masonry (Concrete Work)		6.1	6.5	6.9	7.2	7.6	8.0	8.3	8.7	9.1
Masseur/Masseuse (Standing)		3.5	3.7	3.9	4.1	4.3	4.6	4.8	5.0	5.2
Motocross		3.5	3.7	3.9	4.1	4.3	4.6	4.8	5.0	5.2
Motor Scooter/Cycle		2.2	2.3	2.5	2.6	2.7	2.8	3.0	3.1	3.2
Moving Objects										
Furniture		5.3	5.6	5.9	6.2	6.5	6.8	7.1	7.5	7.8
Heavy objects, more than 75 lb (desks, moving-van work)		6.1	6.5	6.9	7.2	7.6	8.0	8.3	8.7	9.1
Household items in boxes		6.1	6.5	6.9	7.2	7.6	8.0	8.3	8.7	9.1
Household items in boxes up stairs		7.9	8.3	8.8	9.3	9.8	10.2	10.7	11.2	11.7
Ice house (set up/drill holes)		5.3	5.6	5.9	6.2	6.5	6.8	7.1	7.5	7.8
Mowing Lawn										
Riding mower		2.2	2.3	2.5	2.6	2.7	2.8	3.0	3.1	3.2
Manual mower		5.3	5.6	5.9	6.2	6.5	6.8	7.1	7.5	7.8
Push power mower		3.9	4.2	4.4	4.6	4.9	5.1	5.4	5.6	5.8
Office: General										
Doing your own copying, toe lifts while waiting		1.6	1.7	1.8	1.9	2.0	2.1	2.2	2.3	2.4
Going out to lunch (brisk walk to store or restaurant)		2.6	2.8	2.9	3.1	3.2	3.4	3.5	3.7	3.8
Hand-delivering memo		1.8	1.9	2.0	2.1	2.2	2.3	2.4	2.6	2.7
Moving both hands in small circles simultaneously		1.5	1.6	1.7	1.8	1.9	2.0	2.0	2.1	2.2
Swirling computer mouse in circles		1.1	1.2	1.2	1.3	1.4	1.4	1.5	1.6	1.6
Using stairs (down one flight)		2.6	2.8	2.9	3.1	3.2	3.4	3.5	3.7	3.8
Using stairs (up one flight)		7.0	7.4	7.8	8.3	8.7	9.1	9.5	9.9	10.4
Walking while brainstorming (slow walk)		2.2	2.3	2.5	2.6	2.7	2.9	3.0	3.1	3.3
Office: In Chair										
Changing position in chair		1.4	1.5	1.6	1.7	1.7	1.8	1.9	2.0	2.1
Clasping hands on back of head, swinging one elbow forward, then other		1.3	1.4	1.5	1.5	1.6	1.7	1.8	1.8	1.9

Calories Expended by Body Weight

Your Body Weight

77 170	80 176	83 183	86 190	89 196	92 203	95 209	98 216	101 223	104 229	107 236	110 243	113 249	116 256	119 262
9.4	9.8	10.2	10.5	10.9	11.3	11.6	12.0	12.4	12.7	13.1	13.5	13.8	14.2	14.6
5.4	5.6	5.8	6.0	6.2	6.4	6.7	6.9	7.1	7.3	7.5	7.7	7.9	8.1	8.3
5.4	5.6	5.8	6.0	6.2	6.4	6.7	6.9	7.1	7.3	7.5	7.7	7.9	8.1	8.3
3.4	3.5	3.6	3.8	3.9	4.0	4.2	4.3	4.4	4.6	4.7	4.8	4.9	5.1	5.2
8.1	8.4	8.7	9.0	9.3	9.7	10.0	10.3	10.6	10.9	11.2	11.6	11.9	12.2	12.5
9.4	9.8	10.2	10.5	10.9	11.3	11.6	12.0	12.4	12.7	13.1	13.5	13.8	14.2	14.6
9.4	9.8	10.2	10.5	10.9	11.3	11.6	12.0	12.4	12.7	13.1	13.5	13.8	14.2	14.6
12.1	12.6	13.1	13.5	14.0	14.5	15.0	15.4	15.9	16.4	16.9	17.3	17.8	18.3	18.7
8.1	8.4	8.7	9.0	9.3	9.7	10.0	10.3	10.6	10.9	11.2	11.6	11.9	12.2	12.5
3.4	3.5	3.6	3.8	3.9	4.0	4.2	4.3	4.4	4.6	4.7	4.8	4.9	5.1	5.2
8.1	8.4	8.7	9.0	9.3	9.7	10.0	10.3	10.6	10.9	11.2	11.6	11.9	12.2	12.5
6.1	6.3	6.5	6.8	7.0	7.2	7.5	7.7	8.0	8.2	8.4	8.7	8.9	9.1	9.4
2.5	2.6	2.7	2.8	2.8	2.9	3.0	3.1	3.2	3.3	3.4	3.5	3.6	3.7	3.8
4.0	4.2	4.3	4.5	4.6	4.8	4.9	5.1	5.3	5.4	5.6	5.7	5.9	6.0	6.2
2.8	2.9	3.0	3.1	3.2	3.3	3.4	3.5	3.6	3.7	3.9	4.0	4.1	4.2	4.3
2.3	2.4	2.5	2.6	2.7	2.8	2.9	2.9	3.0	3.1	3.2	3.3	3.4	3.5	3.6
1.7	1.8	1.8	1.9	2.0	2.0	2.1	2.2	2.2	2.3	2.4	2.4	2.5	2.6	2.6
4.0	4.2	4.3	4.5	4.6	4.8	4.9	5.1	5.3	5.4	5.6	5.7	5.9	6.0	6.2
10.8	11.2	11.6	12.0	12.5	12.9	13.3	13.7	14.1	14.6	15.0	15.4	15.8	16.2	16.7
3.4	3.5	3.7	3.8	3.9	4.0	4.2	4.3	4.4	4.6	4.7	4.8	5.0	5.1	5.2
2.2	2.2	2.3	2.4	2.5	2.6	2.7	2.7	2.8	2.9	3.0	3.1	3.2	3.2	3.3
2.0	2.1	2.2	2.2	2.3	2.4	2.5	2.5	2.6	2.7	2.8	2.9	2.9	3.0	3.1

Calories Expended by Body Weight

		Your Body Weight								
Activity	**kg** **lb**	**50** **110**	**53** **117**	**56** **123**	**59** **130**	**62** **137**	**65** **143**	**68** **150**	**71** **157**	**74** **163**
Office: In Chair (cont.)										
Crossing and uncrossing legs		1.7	1.8	1.9	2.0	2.1	2.2	2.3	2.4	2.5
Crossing arms, bringing hands down to hips		1.3	1.4	1.5	1.5	1.6	1.7	1.8	1.8	1.9
Elbows on arm rest, lifting one forearm, then other		1.2	1.3	1.3	1.4	1.5	1.6	1.6	1.7	1.8
Holding arms parallel to floor, thrusting one forward and back, repeating with other		2.2	2.3	2.5	2.6	2.7	2.9	3.0	3.1	3.3
Holding arms straight out from sides, rotating forward, backward		1.4	1.5	1.6	1.7	1.7	1.8	1.9	2.0	2.1
Humming loudly		1.0	1.1	1.1	1.2	1.2	1.3	1.4	1.4	1.5
Lifting paperweight or book		1.4	1.5	1.6	1.7	1.7	1.8	1.9	2.0	2.1
Pressing empty stapler to music		1.3	1.4	1.5	1.5	1.6	1.7	1.8	1.8	1.9
Pulling stomach in and out		1.0	1.1	1.1	1.2	1.2	1.3	1.4	1.4	1.5
Pumping foot-pedal under desk		2.5	2.7	2.8	3.0	3.1	3.3	3.4	3.6	3.7
Pushing one foot, then other, against a immovable object		1.6	1.7	1.8	1.9	2.0	2.1	2.2	2.3	2.4
Reaching hand high as you can, low as you can, alternating hands		1.6	1.7	1.8	1.9	2.0	2.1	2.2	2.3	2.4
Rocking chair back and forth		1.4	1.5	1.6	1.7	1.7	1.8	1.9	2.0	2.1
Rocking chair sideways		1.4	1.5	1.6	1.7	1.7	1.8	1.9	2.0	2.1
Rolling chair back and forth, side to side		1.5	1.6	1.7	1.8	1.9	2.0	2.0	2.1	2.2
Shrugging shoulders		1.1	1.2	1.2	1.3	1.4	1.4	1.5	1.6	1.6
Snapping fingers, tapping feet to music		1.5	1.6	1.7	1.8	1.9	2.0	2.0	2.1	2.2
Squeezing soccer ball or volleyball between knees		1.3	1.4	1.5	1.5	1.6	1.7	1.8	1.8	1.9
Squirming		1.1	1.2	1.2	1.3	1.4	1.4	1.5	1.6	1.6
Standing up halfway, sitting down		1.9	2.0	2.1	2.2	2.4	2.5	2.6	2.7	2.8
Stretching rubber band between fingers		1.0	1.1	1.1	1.2	1.2	1.3	1.4	1.4	1.5
Turning head from one side to other, moving head in circular motion		1.2	1.3	1.3	1.4	1.5	1.6	1.6	1.7	1.8
Twirling pencil		1.1	1.2	1.2	1.3	1.4	1.4	1.5	1.6	1.6

Calories Expended by Body Weight

Your Body Weight

| 77 | 80 | 83 | 86 | 89 | 92 | 95 | 98 | 101 | 104 | 107 | 110 | 113 | 116 | 119 |
170	176	183	190	196	203	209	216	223	229	236	243	249	256	262
2.6	2.7	2.8	2.9	3.0	3.1	3.2	3.3	3.4	3.5	3.6	3.7	3.8	3.9	4.0
2.0	2.1	2.2	2.2	2.3	2.4	2.5	2.5	2.6	2.7	2.8	2.9	2.9	3.0	3.1
1.8	1.9	2.0	2.1	2.1	2.2	2.3	2.4	2.4	2.5	2.6	2.6	2.7	2.8	2.9
3.4	3.5	3.7	3.8	3.9	4.0	4.2	4.3	4.4	4.6	4.7	4.8	5.0	5.1	5.2
2.2	2.2	2.3	2.4	2.5	2.6	2.7	2.7	2.8	2.9	3.0	3.1	3.2	3.2	3.3
1.5	1.6	1.7	1.7	1.8	1.8	1.9	2.0	2.0	2.1	2.1	2.2	2.3	2.3	2.4
2.2	2.2	2.3	2.4	2.5	2.6	2.7	2.7	2.8	2.9	3.0	3.1	3.2	3.2	3.3
2.0	2.1	2.2	2.2	2.3	2.4	2.5	2.5	2.6	2.7	2.8	2.9	2.9	3.0	3.1
1.5	1.6	1.7	1.7	1.8	1.8	1.9	2.0	2.0	2.1	2.1	2.2	2.3	2.3	2.4
3.9	4.0	4.2	4.3	4.5	4.6	4.8	4.9	5.1	5.2	5.4	5.5	5.7	5.8	6.0
2.5	2.6	2.7	2.8	2.8	2.9	3.0	3.1	3.2	3.3	3.4	3.5	3.6	3.7	3.8
2.5	2.6	2.7	2.8	2.8	2.9	3.0	3.1	3.2	3.3	3.4	3.5	3.6	3.7	3.8
2.2	2.2	2.3	2.4	2.5	2.6	2.7	2.7	2.8	2.9	3.0	3.1	3.2	3.2	3.3
2.2	2.2	2.3	2.4	2.5	2.6	2.7	2.7	2.8	2.9	3.0	3.1	3.2	3.2	3.3
2.3	2.4	2.5	2.6	2.7	2.8	2.9	2.9	3.0	3.1	3.2	3.3	3.4	3.5	3.6
1.7	1.8	1.8	1.9	2.0	2.0	2.1	2.2	2.2	2.3	2.4	2.4	2.5	2.6	2.6
2.3	2.4	2.5	2.6	2.7	2.8	2.9	2.9	3.0	3.1	3.2	3.3	3.4	3.5	3.6
2.0	2.1	2.2	2.2	2.3	2.4	2.5	2.5	2.6	2.7	2.8	2.9	2.9	3.0	3.1
1.7	1.8	1.8	1.9	2.0	2.0	2.1	2.2	2.2	2.3	2.4	2.4	2.5	2.6	2.6
2.9	3.0	3.2	3.3	3.4	3.5	3.6	3.7	3.8	4.0	4.1	4.2	4.3	4.4	4.5
1.5	1.6	1.7	1.7	1.8	1.8	1.9	2.0	2.0	2.1	2.1	2.2	2.3	2.3	2.4
1.8	1.9	2.0	2.1	2.1	2.2	2.3	2.4	2.4	2.5	2.6	2.6	2.7	2.8	2.9
1.7	1.8	1.8	1.9	2.0	2.0	2.1	2.2	2.2	2.3	2.4	2.4	2.5	2.6	2.6

Calories Expended by Body Weight

Your Body Weight

Activity	kg lb	50 110	53 117	56 123	59 130	62 137	65 143	68 150	71 157	74 163
Office: On the Phone (Standing)										
Holding free arm down straight, making windmill-like circles, alternating arms		1.6	1.7	1.8	1.9	2.0	2.1	2.2	2.3	2.4
Lifting feet off floor		1.4	1.5	1.6	1.7	1.7	1.8	1.9	2.0	2.1
Lifting feet up and down as if walking		1.6	1.7	1.8	1.9	2.0	2.1	2.2	2.3	2.4
Rolling rubber ball on desk, flipping in air		1.2	1.3	1.3	1.4	1.5	1.6	1.6	1.7	1.8
Squeezing piece of rubber or hand grip		1.5	1.6	1.7	1.8	1.9	2.0	2.0	2.1	2.2
Talking with hands		1.5	1.6	1.7	1.8	1.9	2.0	2.0	2.1	2.2
Using hand-held dexterity game		1.3	1.4	1.5	1.5	1.6	1.7	1.8	1.8	1.9
Waving free arm in front of face, alternating arms		1.5	1.6	1.7	1.8	1.9	2.0	2.0	2.1	2.2
Outside the House: Chores and Shopping										
Carrying grocery bags to car (heavy bags in both arms)		6.0	6.4	6.7	7.1	7.4	7.8	8.2	8.5	8.9
Helping older people reach items		1.8	1.9	2.0	2.1	2.2	2.3	2.4	2.6	2.7
Lifting packages up and down		3.3	3.5	3.7	3.9	4.1	4.3	4.5	4.7	4.9
Mall walking, average pace (some stair climbing)		2.9	3.1	3.2	3.4	3.6	3.8	3.9	4.1	4.3
Mall walking, brisk pace (some stair climbing)		3.7	3.9	4.1	4.4	4.6	4.8	5.0	5.3	5.5
Pushing heavy shopping cart		3.4	3.6	3.8	4.0	4.2	4.4	4.6	4.8	5.0
Walking to store: extremely slow (2 mph)		2.2	2.3	2.5	2.6	2.7	2.9	3.0	3.1	3.3
Walking to store: average pace (2.5 mph)		2.6	2.8	2.9	3.1	3.2	3.4	3.5	3.7	3.8
Walking to store: quick pace (3.0 mph)		3.1	3.3	3.5	3.7	3.8	4.0	4.2	4.4	4.6
Walking to store: brisk pace (4.0 mph)		3.5	3.7	3.9	4.1	4.3	4.6	4.8	5.0	5.2
Walking to store: very brisk pace (4.5 mph)		3.9	4.1	4.4	4.6	4.8	5.1	5.3	5.5	5.8
Outside the House: Miscellaneous										
Browsing in book store		1.4	1.5	1.6	1.7	1.7	1.8	1.9	2.0	2.1
Church: collecting contributions		1.4	1.5	1.6	1.7	1.7	1.8	1.9	2.0	2.1

Calories Expended by Body Weight

Your Body Weight

77 170	80 176	83 183	86 190	89 196	92 203	95 209	98 216	101 223	104 229	107 236	110 243	113 249	116 256	119 262
2.5	2.6	2.7	2.8	2.8	2.9	3.0	3.1	3.2	3.3	3.4	3.5	3.6	3.7	3.8
2.2	2.2	2.3	2.4	2.5	2.6	2.7	2.7	2.8	2.9	3.0	3.1	3.2	3.2	3.3
2.5	2.6	2.7	2.8	2.8	2.9	3.0	3.1	3.2	3.3	3.4	3.5	3.6	3.7	3.8
1.8	1.9	2.0	2.1	2.1	2.2	2.3	2.4	2.4	2.5	2.6	2.6	2.7	2.8	2.9
2.3	2.4	2.5	2.6	2.7	2.8	2.9	2.9	3.0	3.1	3.2	3.3	3.4	3.5	3.6
2.3	2.4	2.5	2.6	2.7	2.8	2.9	2.9	3.0	3.1	3.2	3.3	3.4	3.5	3.6
2.0	2.1	2.2	2.2	2.3	2.4	2.5	2.5	2.6	2.7	2.8	2.9	2.9	3.0	3.1
2.3	2.4	2.5	2.6	2.7	2.8	2.9	2.9	3.0	3.1	3.2	3.3	3.4	3.5	3.6
9.2	9.6	10.0	10.3	10.7	11.0	11.4	11.8	12.1	12.5	12.8	13.2	13.6	13.9	14.3
2.8	2.9	3.0	3.1	3.2	3.3	3.4	3.5	3.6	3.7	3.9	4.0	4.1	4.2	4.3
5.1	5.3	5.5	5.7	5.9	6.1	6.3	6.5	6.7	6.9	7.1	7.3	7.5	7.7	7.9
4.5	4.6	4.8	5.0	5.2	5.3	5.5	5.7	5.9	6.0	6.2	6.4	6.6	6.7	6.9
5.7	5.9	6.1	6.4	6.6	6.8	7.0	7.3	7.5	7.7	7.9	8.1	8.4	8.6	8.8
5.2	5.4	5.6	5.8	6.1	6.3	6.5	6.7	6.9	7.1	7.3	7.5	7.7	7.9	8.1
3.4	3.5	3.7	3.8	3.9	4.0	4.2	4.3	4.4	4.6	4.7	4.8	5.0	5.1	5.2
4.0	4.2	4.3	4.5	4.6	4.8	4.9	5.1	5.3	5.4	5.6	5.7	5.9	6.0	6.2
4.8	5.0	5.1	5.3	5.5	5.7	5.9	6.1	6.3	6.4	6.6	6.8	7.0	7.2	7.4
5.4	5.6	5.8	6.0	6.2	6.4	6.7	6.9	7.1	7.3	7.5	7.7	7.9	8.1	8.3
6.0	6.2	6.5	6.7	6.9	7.2	7.4	7.6	7.9	8.1	8.3	8.6	8.8	9.0	9.3
2.2	2.2	2.3	2.4	2.5	2.6	2.7	2.7	2.8	2.9	3.0	3.1	3.2	3.2	3.3
2.2	2.2	2.3	2.4	2.5	2.6	2.7	2.7	2.8	2.9	3.0	3.1	3.2	3.2	3.3

Calories Expended by Body Weight

	Your Body Weight								
Activity	**kg 50** **lb 110**	**53** **117**	**56** **123**	**59** **130**	**62** **137**	**65** **143**	**68** **150**	**71** **157**	**74** **163**
Outside the House: Miscellaneous (cont.)									
Church: painting and doing repairs	3.9	4.1	4.4	4.6	4.8	5.1	5.3	5.5	5.8
Church: ushering	1.1	1.2	1.2	1.3	1.4	1.4	1.5	1.6	1.6
Commuter calisthenics: stretches	1.3	1.4	1.5	1.5	1.6	1.7	1.8	1.8	1.9
Commuter calisthenics: tummy tucks	1.1	1.2	1.2	1.3	1.4	1.4	1.5	1.6	1.6
Doing lifting chores for older neighbor	2.5	2.7	2.8	3.0	3.1	3.3	3.4	3.6	3.7
Lifting legs up and down while waiting for streetlight	2.1	2.2	2.4	2.5	2.6	2.7	2.9	3.0	3.1
Lunging as if fencing	5.0	5.3	5.6	5.9	6.2	6.5	6.8	7.1	7.4
Playing Frisbee with dog	2.4	2.5	2.7	2.8	3.0	3.1	3.3	3.4	3.6
Raking leaves	3.5	3.7	3.9	4.1	4.3	4.6	4.8	5.0	5.2
Shoveling snow	5.3	5.6	5.9	6.3	6.6	6.9	7.2	7.5	7.8
Snowball fight	4.8	5.1	5.4	5.7	6.0	6.2	6.5	6.8	7.1
Waiting on line: rocking back and forth	1.8	1.9	2.0	2.1	2.2	2.3	2.4	2.6	2.7
Waiting on line: shifting weight from foot to foot	1.6	1.7	1.8	1.9	2.0	2.1	2.2	2.3	2.4
Waiting on line: swinging arms	2.0	2.1	2.2	2.4	2.5	2.6	2.7	2.8	3.0
Waiting on line: toe lifts	1.5	1.6	1.7	1.8	1.9	2.0	2.0	2.1	2.2
Walking briskly with 1 lb weights on wrists	3.9	4.1	4.4	4.6	4.8	5.1	5.3	5.5	5.8
Walking up or down escalator	1.7	1.8	1.9	2.0	2.1	2.2	2.3	2.4	2.5
Washing car	3.9	4.1	4.4	4.6	4.8	5.1	5.3	5.5	5.8
Radio Broadcaster	1.5	1.6	1.7	1.8	1.8	1.9	2.0	2.1	2.2
Racquetball									
Casual, general	6.1	6.5	6.9	7.2	7.6	8.0	8.3	8.7	9.1
Competition	9.5	10.0	10.6	11.2	11.7	12.3	12.9	13.4	14.0
Rebound Exercise (Mini-Trampoline)									
120 foot-strikes/min., arm-pumping, holding 1 lb hand weights, 3 ft. jump	10.0	10.6	11.2	11.8	12.4	13.0	13.6	14.2	14.8
120 foot-strikes/min., arm-pumping, holding 1 lb hand weights, 2 ft. jump	8.7	9.2	9.7	10.3	10.8	11.3	11.8	12.4	12.9

Calories Expended by Body Weight

Your Body Weight

77 170	80 176	83 183	86 190	89 196	92 203	95 209	98 216	101 223	104 229	107 236	110 243	113 249	116 256	119 262
6.0	6.2	6.5	6.7	6.9	7.2	7.4	7.6	7.9	8.1	8.3	8.6	8.8	9.0	9.3
1.7	1.8	1.8	1.9	2.0	2.0	2.1	2.2	2.2	2.3	2.4	2.4	2.5	2.6	2.6
2.0	2.1	2.2	2.2	2.3	2.4	2.5	2.5	2.6	2.7	2.8	2.9	2.9	3.0	3.1
1.7	1.8	1.8	1.9	2.0	2.0	2.1	2.2	2.2	2.3	2.4	2.4	2.5	2.6	2.6
3.9	4.0	4.2	4.3	4.5	4.6	4.8	4.9	5.1	5.2	5.4	5.5	5.7	5.8	6.0
3.2	3.4	3.5	3.6	3.7	3.9	4.0	4.1	4.2	4.4	4.5	4.6	4.7	4.9	5.0
7.7	8.0	8.3	8.6	8.9	9.2	9.5	9.8	10.1	10.4	10.7	11.0	11.3	11.6	11.9
3.7	3.8	4.0	4.1	4.3	4.4	4.6	4.7	4.8	5.0	5.1	5.3	5.4	5.6	5.7
5.4	5.6	5.8	6.0	6.2	6.4	6.7	6.9	7.1	7.3	7.5	7.7	7.9	8.1	8.3
8.2	8.5	8.8	9.1	9.4	9.8	10.1	10.4	10.7	11.0	11.3	11.7	12.0	12.3	12.6
7.4	7.7	8.0	8.3	8.5	8.8	9.1	9.4	9.7	10.0	10.3	10.6	10.8	11.1	11.4
2.8	2.9	3.0	3.1	3.2	3.3	3.4	3.5	3.6	3.7	3.9	4.0	4.1	4.2	4.3
2.5	2.6	2.7	2.8	2.8	2.9	3.0	3.1	3.2	3.3	3.4	3.5	3.6	3.7	3.8
3.1	3.2	3.3	3.4	3.6	3.7	3.8	3.9	4.0	4.2	4.3	4.4	4.5	4.6	4.8
2.3	2.4	2.5	2.6	2.7	2.8	2.9	2.9	3.0	3.1	3.2	3.3	3.4	3.5	3.6
6.0	6.2	6.5	6.7	6.9	7.2	7.4	7.6	7.9	8.1	8.3	8.6	8.8	9.0	9.3
2.6	2.7	2.8	2.9	3.0	3.1	3.2	3.3	3.4	3.5	3.6	3.7	3.8	3.9	4.0
6.0	6.2	6.5	6.7	6.9	7.2	7.4	7.6	7.9	8.1	8.3	8.6	8.8	9.0	9.3
2.3	2.4	2.5	2.6	2.6	2.7	2.8	2.9	3.0	3.1	3.2	3.3	3.4	3.5	3.5
9.4	9.8	10.2	10.5	10.9	11.3	11.6	12.0	12.4	12.7	13.1	13.5	13.8	14.2	14.6
14.6	15.1	15.7	16.3	16.8	17.4	18.0	18.5	19.1	19.7	20.2	20.8	21.4	21.9	22.5
15.4	16.0	16.6	17.2	17.8	18.4	19.0	19.6	20.1	20.7	21.3	21.9	22.5	23.1	23.7
13.4	13.9	14.4	15.0	15.5	16.0	16.5	17.0	17.6	18.1	18.6	19.1	19.7	20.2	20.7

Calories Expended by Body Weight

Your Body Weight

Activity	kg 50 lb 110	53 117	56 123	59 130	62 137	65 143	68 150	71 157	74 163
Rebound Exercise (Mini-Trampoline) (cont.)									
120 foot-strikes/min., arm-pumping, holding 3 lb hand weights, 3 ft. jump	11.0	11.6	12.3	12.9	13.6	14.3	14.9	15.6	16.2
120 foot-strikes/min., arm-pumping, holding 3 lb hand weights, 2 ft. jump	9.5	10.0	10.6	11.2	11.7	12.3	12.9	13.4	14.0
120 foot-strikes/min., no arm-pumping, weights, or jumping	6.9	7.3	7.7	8.1	8.5	8.9	9.4	9.8	10.2
Reclining									
Lying quietly (watching TV, reading in bed)	0.9	0.9	1.0	1.1	1.1	1.2	1.2	1.3	1.3
Reading	0.9	0.9	1.0	1.0	1.1	1.1	1.2	1.3	1.3
Talking	0.9	0.9	1.0	1.1	1.1	1.2	1.2	1.3	1.3
Typing	0.9	1.0	1.0	1.1	1.1	1.2	1.2	1.3	1.3
Recreation									
Brisk walking on hard beach sand	3.1	3.3	3.5	3.7	3.8	4.0	4.2	4.4	4.6
Brisk walking on soft beach sand	4.3	4.6	4.8	5.1	5.3	5.6	5.8	6.1	6.4
Brisk walking on soft, wet beach sand	4.5	4.8	5.0	5.3	5.6	5.9	6.1	6.4	6.7
Dancing (ballet, modern, swing, twist, lambada)	5.3	5.6	5.9	6.3	6.6	6.9	7.2	7.5	7.8
Dancing (belly dancing)	5.4	5.7	6.0	6.4	6.7	7.0	7.3	7.7	8.0
Dancing (big band, rock 'n' roll)	4.2	4.5	4.7	5.0	5.2	5.5	5.7	6.0	6.2
Flying a kite (standing)	2.2	2.3	2.5	2.6	2.7	2.9	3.0	3.1	3.3
Flying a kite (standing, walking briskly)	3.3	3.5	3.7	3.9	4.1	4.3	4.5	4.7	4.9
Flying a kite (standing, walking slowly)	2.8	3.0	3.1	3.3	3.5	3.6	3.8	4.0	4.1
Hearty belly-laughing	1.5	1.6	1.7	1.8	1.9	2.0	2.0	2.1	2.2
Knitting	1.3	1.4	1.5	1.5	1.6	1.7	1.8	1.8	1.9
Resistance Exercise Training—Circuit									
General workout (machines)	7.0	7.4	7.8	8.3	8.7	9.1	9.5	9.9	10.4
Universal gym, 10 station (30 sec. exercise, 30 sec. rest), 15–18 reps/station (40% of max strength), men	4.8	5.1	5.4	5.7	6.0	6.3	6.6	6.8	7.1

Calories Expended by Body Weight

Your Body Weight

77 170	80 176	83 183	86 190	89 196	92 203	95 209	98 216	101 223	104 229	107 236	110 243	113 249	116 256	119 262
16.9	17.6	18.2	18.9	19.5	20.2	20.8	21.5	22.2	22.8	23.5	24.1	24.8	25.5	26.1
14.6	15.1	15.7	16.3	16.8	17.4	18.0	18.5	19.1	19.7	20.2	20.8	21.4	21.9	22.5
10.6	11.0	11.4	11.8	12.2	12.7	13.1	13.5	13.9	14.3	14.7	15.1	15.5	16.0	16.4
1.4	1.4	1.5	1.5	1.6	1.6	1.7	1.7	1.8	1.9	1.9	2.0	2.0	2.1	2.1
1.4	1.4	1.5	1.5	1.6	1.6	1.7	1.7	1.8	1.8	1.9	1.9	2.0	2.1	2.1
1.4	1.4	1.5	1.5	1.6	1.6	1.7	1.7	1.8	1.9	1.9	2.0	2.0	2.1	2.1
1.4	1.5	1.5	1.6	1.6	1.7	1.7	1.8	1.8	1.9	1.9	2.0	2.1	2.1	2.2
4.8	5.0	5.1	5.3	5.5	5.7	5.9	6.1	6.3	6.4	6.6	6.8	7.0	7.2	7.4
6.6	6.9	7.1	7.4	7.7	7.9	8.2	8.4	8.7	8.9	9.2	9.5	9.7	10.0	10.2
6.9	7.2	7.5	7.7	8.0	8.3	8.6	8.8	9.1	9.4	9.6	9.9	10.2	10.4	10.7
8.2	8.5	8.8	9.1	9.4	9.8	10.1	10.4	10.7	11.0	11.3	11.7	12.0	12.3	12.6
8.3	8.6	9.0	9.3	9.6	9.9	10.3	10.6	10.9	11.2	11.6	11.9	12.2	12.5	12.9
6.5	6.7	7.0	7.2	7.5	7.7	8.0	8.2	8.5	8.7	9.0	9.2	9.5	9.7	10.0
3.4	3.5	3.7	3.8	3.9	4.0	4.2	4.3	4.4	4.6	4.7	4.8	5.0	5.1	5.2
5.1	5.3	5.5	5.7	5.9	6.1	6.3	6.5	6.7	6.9	7.1	7.3	7.5	7.7	7.9
4.3	4.5	4.6	4.8	5.0	5.2	5.3	5.5	5.7	5.8	6.0	6.2	6.3	6.5	6.7
2.3	2.4	2.5	2.6	2.7	2.8	2.9	2.9	3.0	3.1	3.2	3.3	3.4	3.5	3.6
2.0	2.1	2.2	2.2	2.3	2.4	2.5	2.5	2.6	2.7	2.8	2.9	2.9	3.0	3.1
10.8	11.2	11.6	12.0	12.5	12.9	13.3	13.7	14.1	14.6	15.0	15.4	15.8	16.2	16.7
7.4	7.7	8.0	8.3	8.6	8.9	9.2	9.4	9.7	10.0	10.3	10.6	10.9	11.2	11.5

Calories Expended by Body Weight

Your Body Weight

Activity	kg 50 lb 110	53 117	56 123	59 130	62 137	65 143	68 150	71 157	74 163
Resistance Exercise Training—Circuit (cont.)									
Universal gym, 10 station (30 sec. exercise, 30 sec. rest), 15–18 reps/station (40% of max strength), women	4.3	4.5	4.8	5.0	5.3	5.5	5.8	6.1	6.3
Resistance Exercise Training—Hydra-Fitness+A522									
9 min. circuit (chest press/pull, shoulder press/pull, leg extension/flexion), exercise: rest interval = 1:1, total of 111 reps	6.5	6.9	7.3	7.7	8.1	8.5	8.9	9.2	9.6
9 min. circuit (chest press/pull, shoulder press/pull, leg extension/flexion), exercise:rest interval = 1:2, total of 78 reps	5.7	6.0	6.4	6.7	7.0	7.4	7.7	8.1	8.4
9 min. circuit (chest press/pull, shoulder press/pull, leg extension/flexion), exercise: rest interval = 2:1, total of 141 reps	6.6	7.0	7.4	7.8	8.2	8.6	9.0	9.4	9.8
Behind-neck press, 7 reps	4.8	5.1	5.4	5.7	6.0	6.3	6.5	6.8	7.1
Behind-neck press, 10 reps	4.7	5.0	5.2	5.5	5.8	6.1	6.4	6.6	6.9
Behind-neck press, 14 reps	4.5	4.8	5.0	5.3	5.6	5.8	6.1	6.4	6.6
Bench press, 7 reps	5.3	5.6	6.0	6.3	6.6	6.9	7.2	7.6	7.9
Bench press, 9 reps	5.0	5.3	5.6	5.9	6.2	6.5	6.8	7.1	7.4
Bench press, 17 reps	5.1	5.4	5.7	6.0	6.3	6.6	6.9	7.3	7.6
Bent-over row, 9 reps	6.7	7.1	7.5	8.0	8.4	8.8	9.2	9.6	10.0
Bent-over row, 11 reps	6.5	6.9	7.3	7.7	8.1	8.5	8.9	9.3	9.7
Bent-over row, 19 reps	6.0	6.3	6.7	7.0	7.4	7.8	8.1	8.5	8.8
Biceps curl, 9 reps	5.5	5.8	6.2	6.5	6.8	7.1	7.5	7.8	8.1
Biceps curl, 11 reps	5.4	5.7	6.1	6.4	6.7	7.0	7.4	7.7	8.0
Biceps curl, 15 reps	5.3	5.7	6.0	6.3	6.6	7.0	7.3	7.6	7.9
27-station circuit, 30 sec. exercise, 30 sec. rest, women	5.6	5.9	6.3	6.6	6.9	7.3	7.6	8.0	8.3
27-station circuit, 30 sec. exercise, 30 sec. rest, men	6.1	6.5	6.9	7.2	7.6	8.0	8.3	8.7	9.1
Leg extension, 15 reps	6.4	6.8	7.2	7.6	7.9	8.3	8.7	9.1	9.5
Leg extension, 18 reps	6.5	6.9	7.3	7.7	8.1	8.5	8.8	9.2	9.6

Calories Expended by Body Weight

Your Body Weight

77 170	80 176	83 183	86 190	89 196	92 203	95 209	98 216	101 223	104 229	107 236	110 243	113 249	116 256	119 262
6.6	6.8	7.1	7.3	7.6	7.8	8.1	8.4	8.6	8.9	9.1	9.4	9.6	9.9	10.1
10.0	10.4	10.8	11.2	11.6	12.0	12.4	12.8	13.2	13.5	13.9	14.3	14.7	15.1	15.5
8.7	9.1	9.4	9.8	10.1	10.4	10.8	11.1	11.5	11.8	12.1	12.5	12.8	13.2	13.5
10.2	10.6	11.0	11.4	11.8	12.2	12.6	13.0	13.4	13.8	14.2	14.6	15.0	15.4	15.8
7.4	7.7	8.0	8.3	8.6	8.9	9.1	9.4	9.7	10.0	10.3	10.6	10.9	11.2	11.5
7.2	7.5	7.8	8.0	8.3	8.6	8.9	9.2	9.4	9.7	10.0	10.3	10.6	10.8	11.1
6.9	7.2	7.5	7.7	8.0	8.3	8.5	8.8	9.1	9.3	9.6	9.9	10.1	10.4	10.7
8.2	8.5	8.8	9.2	9.5	9.8	10.1	10.4	10.7	11.1	11.4	11.7	12.0	12.3	12.7
7.7	8.0	8.3	8.6	8.9	9.2	9.5	9.8	10.1	10.4	10.7	11.0	11.4	11.7	12.0
7.9	8.2	8.5	8.8	9.1	9.4	9.7	10.0	10.3	10.6	10.9	11.2	11.5	11.9	12.2
10.4	10.8	11.2	11.6	12.0	12.4	12.8	13.2	13.6	14.0	14.4	14.8	15.2	15.6	16.0
10.1	10.4	10.8	11.2	11.6	12.0	12.4	12.8	13.2	13.6	14.0	14.4	14.8	15.1	15.5
9.2	9.5	9.9	10.3	10.6	11.0	11.3	11.7	12.1	12.4	12.8	13.1	13.5	13.8	14.2
8.5	8.8	9.1	9.5	9.8	10.1	10.4	10.8	11.1	11.4	11.8	12.1	12.4	12.7	13.1
8.3	8.7	9.0	9.3	9.6	9.9	10.3	10.6	10.9	11.2	11.6	11.9	12.2	12.5	12.9
8.2	8.6	8.9	9.2	9.5	9.8	10.2	10.5	10.8	11.1	11.4	11.8	12.1	12.4	12.7
8.6	9.0	9.3	9.6	10.0	10.3	10.6	11.0	11.3	11.6	12.0	12.3	12.7	13.0	13.3
9.4	9.8	10.2	10.6	10.9	11.3	11.7	12.0	12.4	12.8	13.1	13.5	13.9	14.2	14.6
9.9	10.2	10.6	11.0	11.4	11.8	12.2	12.6	12.9	13.3	13.7	14.1	14.5	14.9	15.2
10.0	10.4	10.8	11.2	11.6	12.0	12.4	12.7	13.1	13.5	13.9	14.3	14.7	15.1	15.5

Calories Expended by Body Weight

Your Body Weight

Activity	kg 50 lb 110	53 117	56 123	59 130	62 137	65 143	68 150	71 157	74 163
Resistance Exercise Training—Hydra-Fitness+A522 (cont.)									
Leg extension, 25 reps	4.8	5.0	5.3	5.6	5.9	6.2	6.5	6.7	7.0
Sitting chest press, 20 reps	6.4	6.8	7.2	7.5	7.9	8.3	8.7	9.1	9.5
Sitting leg extension, 18 reps	7.2	7.6	8.0	8.5	8.9	9.3	9.8	10.2	10.6
Sitting shoulder press, 16 reps	6.0	6.4	6.8	7.1	7.5	7.8	8.2	8.6	8.9
Squat, 9 reps	7.2	7.6	8.0	8.5	8.9	9.3	9.8	10.2	10.6
Squat, 11 reps	7.1	7.5	7.9	8.3	8.8	9.2	9.6	10.0	10.5
Squat, 19 reps	6.3	6.6	7.0	7.4	7.8	8.1	8.5	8.9	9.3
Upright row, 7 reps	5.8	6.2	6.5	6.9	7.2	7.6	7.9	8.3	8.6
Upright row, 10 reps	6.1	6.5	6.8	7.2	7.6	7.9	8.3	8.6	9.0
Upright row, 13 reps	5.6	5.9	6.2	6.6	6.9	7.2	7.6	7.9	8.2
Resistance Exercise Training—Nautilus									
12 exercises, 8–12 reps each, 14–19 min. duration	4.1	4.4	4.6	4.9	5.1	5.4	5.6	5.9	6.1
Express circuit, 5 leg exercises (8–10 reps each), 8 arm exercises (8–15 reps each), 1 abdominal exercise performed to muscular failure	4.8	5.1	5.4	5.7	6.0	6.3	6.6	6.9	7.1
Resistance Exercise Training— Universal Gym	6.1	6.5	6.8	7.2	7.6	7.9	8.3	8.6	9.0
Rock Climbing									
Ascending rock	9.6	10.2	10.8	11.4	11.9	12.5	13.1	13.7	14.2
Rappelling	7.0	7.4	7.8	8.3	8.7	9.1	9.5	9.9	10.4
Rock or mountain climbing	7.0	7.4	7.8	8.3	8.7	9.1	9.5	9.9	10.4
Treadwall rock climbing treadmill	7.9	8.4	8.8	9.3	9.8	10.3	10.7	11.2	11.7
Roller Skating									
Inside, rink	5.7	6.0	6.4	6.7	7.1	7.4	7.7	8.1	8.4
Outside, pavement	6.2	6.6	7.0	7.3	7.7	8.1	8.4	8.8	9.2
Roller Skiing									
Diagonal method (5% grade, 8.7 mph)	11.6	12.3	13.0	13.7	14.4	15.1	15.8	16.5	17.2
Double-pole method, trained athletes (8.7 mph)	7.2	7.6	8.0	8.5	8.9	9.3	9.8	10.2	10.6

Calories Expended by Body Weight

Your Body Weight

77 170	80 176	83 183	86 190	89 196	92 203	95 209	98 216	101 223	104 229	107 236	110 243	113 249	116 256	119 262
7.3	7.6	7.9	8.2	8.5	8.7	9.0	9.3	9.6	9.9	10.2	10.5	10.7	11.0	11.3
9.8	10.2	10.6	11.0	11.4	11.8	12.1	12.5	12.9	13.3	13.7	14.1	14.4	14.8	15.2
11.0	11.5	11.9	12.3	12.8	13.2	13.6	14.1	14.5	14.9	15.4	15.8	16.2	16.6	17.1
9.3	9.7	10.0	10.4	10.7	11.1	11.5	11.8	12.2	12.6	12.9	13.3	13.6	14.0	14.4
11.1	11.5	11.9	12.4	12.8	13.2	13.6	14.1	14.5	14.9	15.4	15.8	16.2	16.7	17.1
10.9	11.3	11.7	12.1	12.6	13.0	13.4	13.8	14.3	14.7	15.1	15.5	16.0	16.4	16.8
9.6	10.0	10.4	10.8	11.2	11.5	11.9	12.3	12.7	13.0	13.4	13.8	14.2	14.5	14.9
9.0	9.3	9.7	10.0	10.4	10.7	11.1	11.4	11.8	12.1	12.5	12.8	13.2	13.5	13.8
9.4	9.7	10.1	10.5	10.8	11.2	11.6	11.9	12.3	12.7	13.0	13.4	13.8	14.1	14.5
8.6	8.9	9.2	9.6	9.9	10.2	10.6	10.9	11.2	11.6	11.9	12.2	12.6	12.9	13.2
6.4	6.6	6.9	7.1	7.4	7.6	7.9	8.1	8.4	8.6	8.9	9.1	9.4	9.6	9.9
7.4	7.7	8.0	8.3	8.6	8.9	9.2	9.5	9.8	10.0	10.3	10.6	10.9	11.2	11.5
9.4	9.7	10.1	10.5	10.8	11.2	11.6	11.9	12.3	12.7	13.0	13.4	13.8	14.1	14.5
14.8	15.4	16.0	16.6	17.1	17.7	18.3	18.9	19.4	20.0	20.6	21.2	21.8	22.3	22.9
10.8	11.2	11.6	12.0	12.5	12.9	13.3	13.7	14.1	14.6	15.0	15.4	15.8	16.2	16.7
10.8	11.2	11.6	12.0	12.5	12.9	13.3	13.7	14.1	14.6	15.0	15.4	15.8	16.2	16.7
12.2	12.6	13.1	13.6	14.1	14.5	15.0	15.5	16.0	16.4	16.9	17.4	17.9	18.3	18.8
8.8	9.1	9.4	9.8	10.1	10.5	10.8	11.1	11.5	11.8	12.2	12.5	12.9	13.2	13.5
9.6	9.9	10.3	10.7	11.1	11.4	11.8	12.2	12.5	12.9	13.3	13.7	14.0	14.4	14.8
17.9	18.6	19.3	20.0	20.7	21.4	22.1	22.8	23.5	24.2	24.9	25.6	26.3	27.0	27.7
11.0	11.5	11.9	12.3	12.8	13.2	13.6	14.1	14.5	14.9	15.4	15.8	16.2	16.6	17.1

Calories Expended by Body Weight

Your Body Weight

Activity	kg 50 lb 110	53 117	56 123	59 130	62 137	65 143	68 150	71 157	74 163
Roller Skiing (cont.)									
Double-pole method, trained athletes (11.2 mph)	10.2	10.8	11.4	12.0	12.7	13.3	13.9	14.5	15.1
Double-pole method, long or short poles (2.5 mph)	4.9	5.2	5.5	5.8	6.1	6.4	6.7	7.0	7.3
Double-pole method, long or short poles (4.5 mph)	7.1	7.5	7.9	8.4	8.8	9.2	9.7	10.1	10.5
Double-pole method, long or short poles (6.5 mph)	9.1	9.7	10.2	10.8	11.3	11.9	12.4	12.9	13.5
Kick double-pole method, trained athletes (8.7 mph)	8.1	8.6	9.1	9.6	10.1	10.6	11.1	11.5	12.0
Kick double-pole method, trained athletes (11.2 mph)	11.5	12.2	12.9	13.6	14.3	14.9	15.6	16.3	17.0
Running method, on asphalt (5% grade, 8.7 mph)	11.8	12.5	13.2	13.9	14.7	15.4	16.1	16.8	17.5
Ski imitation with poles, on asphalt (5% grade, 6.9 mph)	12.3	13.1	13.8	14.6	15.3	16.0	16.8	17.5	18.3
V-Skate double-pole method, on asphalt (5% grade, 5.4 mph)	8.3	8.8	9.3	9.8	10.3	10.8	11.3	11.8	12.3
V-Skate double-pole method, on asphalt (5% grade, 6.5 mph)	9.8	10.4	11.0	11.6	12.2	12.7	13.3	13.9	14.5
V-Skate double-pole method, on asphalt (5% grade, 7.4 mph)	10.9	11.6	12.3	12.9	13.6	14.2	14.9	15.5	16.2
V-Skate skate method, on asphalt (5% grade, 5.4 mph)	8.9	9.5	10.0	10.5	11.1	11.6	12.1	12.7	13.2
V-Skate skate method, on asphalt (5% grade, 6.5 mph)	10.5	11.1	11.8	12.4	13.0	13.7	14.3	14.9	15.5
V-Skate skate method, on asphalt (5% grade, 7.4 mph)	11.9	12.6	13.3	14.0	14.8	15.5	16.2	16.9	17.6
V-Skate skate method, trained athletes (11.2 mph)	11.3	12.0	12.7	13.4	14.0	14.7	15.4	16.1	16.8
V-Skate skate method, trained athletes (8.7 mph)	8.5	9.0	9.5	10.0	10.5	11.0	11.5	12.0	12.5
V-Skate skate method, highly trained athletes (11.2 mph)	13.9	14.7	15.6	16.4	17.2	18.1	18.9	19.7	20.6
Roofing									
General	5.3	5.6	5.9	6.2	6.5	6.8	7.1	7.5	7.8
Raking roof with snow rake	3.5	3.7	3.9	4.1	4.3	4.6	4.8	5.0	5.2

Calories Expended by Body Weight

Your Body Weight

77	80	83	86	89	92	95	98	101	104	107	110	113	116	119
170	176	183	190	196	203	209	216	223	229	236	243	249	256	262
15.7	16.3	16.9	17.5	18.2	18.8	19.4	20.0	20.6	21.2	21.8	22.4	23.1	23.7	24.3
7.6	7.9	8.1	8.4	8.7	9.0	9.3	9.6	9.9	10.2	10.5	10.8	11.1	11.4	11.7
10.9	11.4	11.8	12.2	12.6	13.1	13.5	13.9	14.3	14.8	15.2	15.6	16.0	16.5	16.9
14.0	14.6	15.1	15.7	16.2	16.8	17.3	17.9	18.4	19.0	19.5	20.1	20.6	21.2	21.7
12.5	13.0	13.5	14.0	14.5	15.0	15.4	15.9	16.4	16.9	17.4	17.9	18.4	18.9	19.3
17.7	18.4	19.1	19.8	20.5	21.2	21.8	22.5	23.2	23.9	24.6	25.3	26.0	26.7	27.4
18.2	18.9	19.6	20.3	21.0	21.8	22.5	23.2	23.9	24.6	25.3	26.0	26.7	27.4	28.1
19.0	19.7	20.5	21.2	22.0	22.7	23.4	24.2	24.9	25.7	26.4	27.1	27.9	28.6	29.4
12.8	13.3	13.8	14.3	14.8	15.3	15.8	16.3	16.8	17.3	17.8	18.3	18.8	19.3	19.8
15.1	15.7	16.3	16.9	17.4	18.0	18.6	19.2	19.8	20.4	21.0	21.6	22.1	22.7	23.3
16.8	17.5	18.2	18.8	19.5	20.1	20.8	21.4	22.1	22.8	23.4	24.1	24.7	25.4	26.0
13.7	14.3	14.8	15.4	15.9	16.4	17.0	17.5	18.0	18.6	19.1	19.6	20.2	20.7	21.2
16.2	16.8	17.4	18.1	18.7	19.3	20.0	20.6	21.2	21.8	22.5	23.1	23.7	24.4	25.0
18.3	19.0	19.8	20.5	21.2	21.9	22.6	23.3	24.0	24.8	25.5	26.2	26.9	27.6	28.3
17.4	18.1	18.8	19.5	20.2	20.8	21.5	22.2	22.9	23.6	24.2	24.9	25.6	26.3	26.9
13.0	13.5	14.0	14.5	15.0	15.6	16.1	16.6	17.1	17.6	18.1	18.6	19.1	19.6	20.1
21.4	22.2	23.1	23.9	24.7	25.6	26.4	27.2	28.1	28.9	29.7	30.6	31.4	32.2	33.1
8.1	8.4	8.7	9.0	9.3	9.7	10.0	10.3	10.6	10.9	11.2	11.6	11.9	12.2	12.5
5.4	5.6	5.8	6.0	6.2	6.4	6.7	6.9	7.1	7.3	7.5	7.7	7.9	8.1	8.3

			Calories Expended by Body Weight						
				Your Body Weight					
Activity	**kg 50** **lb 110**	**53** **117**	**56** **123**	**59** **130**	**62** **137**	**65** **143**	**68** **150**	**71** **157**	**74** **163**
Rowing—Concept II Rowing Ergometer									
50 watts, men, 16 mph, ages 20–29	3.9	4.1	4.3	4.6	4.8	5.0	5.3	5.5	5.7
50 watts, men, ages 20–29	3.6	3.8	4.1	4.3	4.5	4.7	4.9	5.1	5.4
50 watts, men, ages 30–39	4.0	4.2	4.5	4.7	4.9	5.2	5.4	5.7	5.9
50 watts, men, ages 40–49	3.7	4.0	4.2	4.4	4.6	4.8	5.1	5.3	5.5
50 watts, men, ages 50–59	3.9	4.1	4.3	4.6	4.8	5.0	5.3	5.5	5.7
50 watts, men, age 60+	3.7	4.0	4.2	4.4	4.6	4.8	5.1	5.3	5.5
50 watts, women, 16 mph, ages 20–29	4.0	4.2	4.4	4.7	4.9	5.2	5.4	5.6	5.9
50 watts, women, ages 20–29	3.6	3.8	4.0	4.2	4.4	4.6	4.8	5.0	5.3
50 watts, women, ages 30–39	3.4	3.6	3.8	4.0	4.2	4.4	4.6	4.8	5.0
50 watts, women, ages 40–49	4.2	4.4	4.7	4.9	5.2	5.4	5.7	5.9	6.2
50 watts, women, ages 50–59	3.4	3.6	3.8	4.0	4.2	4.4	4.7	4.9	5.1
60 watts, men, ages 20–29	4.7	5.0	5.3	5.6	5.9	6.2	6.4	6.7	7.0
60 watts, men, ages 30–39	5.3	5.6	5.9	6.3	6.6	6.9	7.2	7.5	7.8
60 watts, men, ages 40–49	5.2	5.5	5.8	6.1	6.4	6.7	7.1	7.4	7.7
60 watts, men, ages 50–59	5.1	5.4	5.7	6.0	6.3	6.6	6.9	7.3	7.6
60 watts, men, age 60+	4.9	5.2	5.5	5.8	6.1	6.4	6.7	6.9	7.2
60 watts, women, ages 20–29	5.0	5.3	5.6	5.9	6.2	6.6	6.9	7.2	7.5
60 watts, women, ages 30–39	5.1	5.4	5.7	6.0	6.3	6.6	6.9	7.2	7.5
60 watts, women, ages 40–49	5.4	5.7	6.0	6.4	6.7	7.0	7.3	7.7	8.0
60 watts, women, ages 50–59	4.5	4.8	5.1	5.3	5.6	5.9	6.1	6.4	6.7
90 watts, men, ages 20–29	5.6	5.9	6.3	6.6	6.9	7.3	7.6	8.0	8.3
90 watts, men, ages 30–39	6.3	6.7	7.1	7.5	7.9	8.2	8.6	9.0	9.4
90 watts, men, ages 40–49	6.2	6.5	6.9	7.3	7.6	8.0	8.4	8.7	9.1
90 watts, men, ages 50–59	6.1	6.5	6.9	7.2	7.6	8.0	8.3	8.7	9.1
90 watts, men, age 60+	5.7	6.0	6.4	6.7	7.0	7.4	7.7	8.1	8.4
90 watts, women, ages 20–29	6.1	6.5	6.9	7.2	7.6	8.0	8.4	8.7	9.1
90 watts, women, ages 30–39	6.1	6.5	6.9	7.2	7.6	8.0	8.4	8.7	9.1
90 watts, women, ages 40–49	6.2	6.6	6.9	7.3	7.7	8.0	8.4	8.8	9.2
90 watts, women, ages 50–59	5.3	5.6	5.9	6.2	6.5	6.8	7.2	7.5	7.8
110 watts, men, ages 20–29	6.8	7.2	7.6	8.1	8.5	8.9	9.3	9.7	10.1
110 watts, men, ages 30–39	7.5	8.0	8.4	8.9	9.3	9.8	10.2	10.7	11.1
110 watts, men, ages 40–49	7.1	7.5	8.0	8.4	8.8	9.3	9.7	10.1	10.5
110 watts, men, ages 50–59	7.1	7.5	8.0	8.4	8.8	9.3	9.7	10.1	10.5
110 watts, men, age 60+	6.3	6.7	7.1	7.5	7.9	8.2	8.6	9.0	9.4

Calories Expended by Body Weight

Your Body Weight

77 170	80 176	83 183	86 190	89 196	92 203	95 209	98 216	101 223	104 229	107 236	110 243	113 249	116 256	119 262
6.0	6.2	6.4	6.7	6.9	7.1	7.3	7.6	7.8	8.0	8.3	8.5	8.7	9.0	9.2
5.6	5.8	6.0	6.2	6.4	6.7	6.9	7.1	7.3	7.5	7.8	8.0	8.2	8.4	8.6
6.1	6.4	6.6	6.9	7.1	7.3	7.6	7.8	8.1	8.3	8.5	8.8	9.0	9.3	9.5
5.7	6.0	6.2	6.4	6.6	6.9	7.1	7.3	7.5	7.8	8.0	8.2	8.4	8.6	8.9
6.0	6.2	6.4	6.7	6.9	7.1	7.4	7.6	7.8	8.1	8.3	8.5	8.8	9.0	9.2
5.7	6.0	6.2	6.4	6.6	6.9	7.1	7.3	7.5	7.8	8.0	8.2	8.4	8.6	8.9
6.1	6.4	6.6	6.8	7.1	7.3	7.5	7.8	8.0	8.3	8.5	8.7	9.0	9.2	9.5
5.5	5.7	5.9	6.1	6.3	6.5	6.7	7.0	7.2	7.4	7.6	7.8	8.0	8.2	8.5
5.2	5.4	5.6	5.8	6.0	6.2	6.4	6.6	6.8	7.0	7.2	7.4	7.6	7.8	8.0
6.4	6.7	6.9	7.2	7.4	7.7	7.9	8.2	8.4	8.7	8.9	9.2	9.4	9.7	9.9
5.3	5.5	5.7	5.9	6.1	6.3	6.5	6.7	6.9	7.1	7.3	7.5	7.7	7.9	8.1
7.3	7.6	7.9	8.2	8.4	8.7	9.0	9.3	9.6	9.9	10.1	10.4	10.7	11.0	11.3
8.2	8.5	8.8	9.1	9.4	9.8	10.1	10.4	10.7	11.0	11.3	11.7	12.0	12.3	12.6
8.0	8.3	8.6	8.9	9.2	9.5	9.9	10.2	10.5	10.8	11.1	11.4	11.7	12.0	12.3
7.9	8.2	8.5	8.8	9.1	9.4	9.7	10.0	10.3	10.6	10.9	11.2	11.5	11.9	12.2
7.5	7.8	8.1	8.4	8.7	9.0	9.3	9.6	9.9	10.2	10.5	10.8	11.1	11.3	11.6
7.8	8.1	8.4	8.7	9.0	9.3	9.6	9.9	10.2	10.5	10.8	11.1	11.4	11.7	12.0
7.8	8.1	8.4	8.7	9.0	9.4	9.7	10.0	10.3	10.6	10.9	11.2	11.5	11.8	12.1
8.3	8.6	9.0	9.3	9.6	9.9	10.3	10.6	10.9	11.2	11.6	11.9	12.2	12.5	12.8
7.0	7.2	7.5	7.8	8.0	8.3	8.6	8.8	9.1	9.4	9.7	9.9	10.2	10.5	10.7
8.6	9.0	9.3	9.6	10.0	10.3	10.6	11.0	11.3	11.6	12.0	12.3	12.7	13.0	13.3
9.8	10.2	10.5	10.9	11.3	11.7	12.1	12.4	12.8	13.2	13.6	14.0	14.3	14.7	15.1
9.5	9.9	10.2	10.6	11.0	11.3	11.7	12.1	12.4	12.8	13.2	13.6	13.9	14.3	14.7
9.4	9.8	10.2	10.5	10.9	11.3	11.6	12.0	12.4	12.7	13.1	13.5	13.8	14.2	14.6
8.7	9.1	9.4	9.8	10.1	10.4	10.8	11.1	11.5	11.8	12.1	12.5	12.8	13.2	13.5
9.5	9.8	10.2	10.6	10.9	11.3	11.7	12.0	12.4	12.8	13.1	13.5	13.9	14.3	14.6
9.5	9.8	10.2	10.6	10.9	11.3	11.7	12.0	12.4	12.8	13.1	13.5	13.9	14.3	14.6
9.5	9.9	10.3	10.6	11.0	11.4	11.8	12.1	12.5	12.9	13.2	13.6	14.0	14.4	14.7
8.1	8.4	8.7	9.1	9.4	9.7	10.0	10.3	10.6	11.0	11.3	11.6	11.9	12.2	12.5
10.5	10.9	11.3	11.7	12.1	12.6	13.0	13.4	13.8	14.2	14.6	15.0	15.4	15.8	16.2
11.6	12.1	12.5	13.0	13.4	13.9	14.3	14.8	15.2	15.7	16.1	16.6	17.0	17.5	17.9
11.0	11.4	11.8	12.3	12.7	13.1	13.5	14.0	14.4	14.8	15.2	15.7	16.1	16.5	17.0
11.0	11.4	11.8	12.3	12.7	13.1	13.5	14.0	14.4	14.8	15.2	15.7	16.1	16.5	17.0
9.8	10.2	10.5	10.9	11.3	11.7	12.1	12.4	12.8	13.2	13.6	14.0	14.3	14.7	15.1

Calories Expended by Body Weight

Your Body Weight

Activity	kg 50 lb 110	53 117	56 123	59 130	62 137	65 143	68 150	71 157	74 163
Rowing—Concept II Rowing Ergometer (cont.)									
110 watts, women, ages 20–29	7.3	7.7	8.2	8.6	9.0	9.5	9.9	10.3	10.8
110 watts, women, ages 30–39	7.3	7.7	8.2	8.6	9.0	9.5	9.9	10.3	10.8
110 watts, women, ages 40–49	6.8	7.3	7.7	8.1	8.5	8.9	9.3	9.7	10.1
125 watts, men, 19.9 mph, ages 20–30	5.6	5.9	6.3	6.6	6.9	7.3	7.6	8.0	8.3
125 watts, women, 19.9 mph, ages 20–30	5.9	6.2	6.6	6.9	7.3	7.6	8.0	8.3	8.7
140 watts, men, ages 20–29	7.9	8.4	8.9	9.4	9.9	10.3	10.8	11.3	11.8
140 watts, men, ages 30–39	8.7	9.3	9.8	10.3	10.8	11.4	11.9	12.4	12.9
140 watts, men, ages 40–49	8.1	8.6	9.1	9.6	10.0	10.5	11.0	11.5	12.0
140 watts, men, ages 50–59	8.0	8.5	9.0	9.5	9.9	10.4	10.9	11.4	11.9
140 watts, men, age 60+	7.2	7.6	8.0	8.5	8.9	9.3	9.7	10.2	10.6
140 watts, women, ages 20–29	8.5	9.0	9.5	10.0	10.5	11.1	11.6	12.1	12.6
140 watts, women, ages 30–39	8.6	9.1	9.6	10.1	10.7	11.2	11.7	12.2	12.7
175 watts, men, 23.6 mph, ages 20–31	8.2	8.7	9.2	9.7	10.2	10.7	11.2	11.6	12.1
175 watts, women, 23.6 mph, ages 20-31	8.7	9.2	9.8	10.3	10.8	11.3	11.9	12.4	12.9
180 watts, men, ages 20–29	9.5	10.1	10.7	11.2	11.8	12.4	12.9	13.5	14.1
180 watts, men, ages 30–39	10.1	10.7	11.3	11.9	12.5	13.1	13.8	14.4	15.0
180 watts, men, ages 40–49	9.3	9.8	10.4	10.9	11.5	12.0	12.6	13.1	13.7
180 watts, men, ages 50–59	9.0	9.5	10.0	10.6	11.1	11.6	12.2	12.7	13.2
210 watts, men, ages 20–29	10.7	11.4	12.0	12.6	13.3	13.9	14.6	15.2	15.9
210 watts, men, ages 30–39	11.7	12.4	13.1	13.8	14.5	15.2	15.9	16.6	17.3
210 watts, men, ages 40–49	10.5	11.2	11.8	12.4	13.1	13.7	14.3	14.9	15.6
250 watts, men, ages 20–29	12.4	13.1	13.8	14.6	15.3	16.1	16.8	17.5	18.3
250 watts, men, ages 30–39	12.7	13.4	14.2	14.9	15.7	16.4	17.2	18.0	18.7
250 watts, men, ages 40–49	12.4	13.2	13.9	14.7	15.4	16.2	16.9	17.6	18.4
78% of max heart rate, men	8.7	9.2	9.7	10.2	10.7	11.2	11.8	12.3	12.8
78% of max heart rate, women	7.1	7.5	8.0	8.4	8.8	9.3	9.7	10.1	10.5
Rowing—Crew									
2.0 to 3.9 mph, light effort, recreational	3.2	3.3	3.5	3.7	3.9	4.1	4.3	4.5	4.7
4.0 to 5.9 mph, moderate effort, recreational	6.5	6.9	7.3	7.6	8.0	8.4	8.8	9.2	9.6
More than 6 mph, vigorous effort, recreational	10.7	11.3	12.0	12.6	13.2	13.9	14.5	15.2	15.8

Calories Expended by Body Weight

Your Body Weight

77 170	80 176	83 183	86 190	89 196	92 203	95 209	98 216	101 223	104 229	107 236	110 243	113 249	116 256	119 262
11.2	11.6	12.1	12.5	13.0	13.4	13.8	14.3	14.7	15.1	15.6	16.0	16.5	16.9	17.3
11.2	11.6	12.1	12.5	13.0	13.4	13.8	14.3	14.7	15.1	15.6	16.0	16.5	16.9	17.3
10.5	10.9	11.4	11.8	12.2	12.6	13.0	13.4	13.8	14.2	14.6	15.1	15.5	15.9	16.3
8.6	9.0	9.3	9.6	10.0	10.3	10.6	11.0	11.3	11.6	12.0	12.3	12.7	13.0	13.3
9.0	9.4	9.7	10.1	10.4	10.8	11.1	11.5	11.8	12.2	12.5	12.9	13.2	13.6	13.9
12.2	12.7	13.2	13.7	14.1	14.6	15.1	15.6	16.0	16.5	17.0	17.5	18.0	18.4	18.9
13.4	14.0	14.5	15.0	15.5	16.1	16.6	17.1	17.6	18.2	18.7	19.2	19.7	20.3	20.8
12.5	13.0	13.4	13.9	14.4	14.9	15.4	15.9	16.3	16.8	17.3	17.8	18.3	18.8	19.3
12.4	12.8	13.3	13.8	14.3	14.8	15.2	15.7	16.2	16.7	17.2	17.7	18.1	18.6	19.1
11.0	11.5	11.9	12.3	12.8	13.2	13.6	14.0	14.5	14.9	15.3	15.8	16.2	16.6	17.1
13.1	13.6	14.1	14.6	15.1	15.6	16.2	16.7	17.2	17.7	18.2	18.7	19.2	19.7	20.2
13.2	13.7	14.3	14.8	15.3	15.8	16.3	16.8	17.4	17.9	18.4	18.9	19.4	19.9	20.5
12.6	13.1	13.6	14.1	14.6	15.1	15.6	16.1	16.6	17.1	17.5	18.0	18.5	19.0	19.5
13.4	14.0	14.5	15.0	15.5	16.1	16.6	17.1	17.6	18.1	18.7	19.2	19.7	20.2	20.8
14.6	15.2	15.8	16.4	16.9	17.5	18.1	18.6	19.2	19.8	20.4	20.9	21.5	22.1	22.6
15.6	16.2	16.8	17.4	18.0	18.6	19.2	19.8	20.4	21.0	21.6	22.3	22.9	23.5	24.1
14.3	14.8	15.4	15.9	16.5	17.0	17.6	18.1	18.7	19.3	19.8	20.4	20.9	21.5	22.0
13.8	14.3	14.9	15.4	15.9	16.5	17.0	17.5	18.1	18.6	19.2	19.7	20.2	20.8	21.3
16.5	17.1	17.8	18.4	19.1	19.7	20.3	21.0	21.6	22.3	22.9	23.6	24.2	24.8	25.5
18.0	18.7	19.4	20.2	20.9	21.6	22.3	23.0	23.7	24.4	25.1	25.8	26.5	27.2	27.9
16.2	16.8	17.5	18.1	18.7	19.4	20.0	20.6	21.3	21.9	22.5	23.2	23.8	24.4	25.1
19.0	19.8	20.5	21.3	22.0	22.7	23.5	24.2	25.0	25.7	26.4	27.2	27.9	28.7	29.4
19.5	20.2	21.0	21.8	22.5	23.3	24.0	24.8	25.6	26.3	27.1	27.8	28.6	29.4	30.1
19.1	19.9	20.6	21.4	22.1	22.9	23.6	24.4	25.1	25.8	26.6	27.3	28.1	28.8	29.6
13.3	13.8	14.4	14.9	15.4	15.9	16.4	17.0	17.5	18.0	18.5	19.0	19.6	20.1	20.6
11.0	11.4	11.8	12.3	12.7	13.1	13.5	14.0	14.4	14.8	15.2	15.7	16.1	16.5	17.0
4.9	5.0	5.2	5.4	5.6	5.8	6.0	6.2	6.4	6.6	6.7	6.9	7.1	7.3	7.5
10.0	10.4	10.7	11.1	11.5	11.9	12.3	12.7	13.1	13.5	13.9	14.2	14.6	15.0	15.4
16.4	17.1	17.7	18.4	19.0	19.6	20.3	20.9	21.6	22.2	22.8	23.5	24.1	24.8	25.4

Calories Expended by Body Weight

Activity	kg 50 lb 110	53 117	56 123	59 130	62 137	65 143	68 150	71 157	74 163
Rowing—Crew (cont.)									
Crew or sculling, competition	11.7	12.4	13.1	13.8	14.5	15.2	15.9	16.6	17.4
General, recreational	3.2	3.4	3.6	3.8	4.0	4.2	4.4	4.6	4.8
Maximal effort	11.2	11.9	12.5	13.2	13.9	14.6	15.2	15.9	16.6
Rowing—Maximal Test									
All-out for 6 min. on rowing ergometer	15.9	16.9	17.8	18.8	19.7	20.7	21.7	22.6	23.6
Concept II	11.2	11.9	12.5	13.2	13.9	14.6	15.2	15.9	16.6
Gjessing Ergo-Row	12.1	12.8	13.6	14.3	15.0	15.7	16.5	17.2	17.9
Hydraulic rower (Hydra-Fitness), 30 cycles/min., 50% of max arm force during rowing, all-out last 2 min.	10.9	11.6	12.3	12.9	13.6	14.2	14.9	15.5	16.2
Hydraulic rower (Hydra-Fitness), 30 cycles/min., 50% max arm force, incremental from setting 1 to 6 (durations of 5, 5, 3, 2, 1 min.)	8.9	9.4	10.0	10.5	11.0	11.6	12.1	12.6	13.2
Mechanical ergometer in rowing tank	13.4	14.2	15.0	15.8	16.6	17.4	18.2	19.0	19.8
Precor 612 rowing ergometer	9.2	9.7	10.3	10.8	11.3	11.9	12.4	13.0	13.5
Rowing—Mechanically Braked Ergometer									
28–32 strokes/min., 1,000 kg·m/min., athletes	10.7	11.3	12.0	12.6	13.3	13.9	14.5	15.2	15.8
28–32 strokes/min., 1,000 kg·m/min., nonathletes	10.1	10.7	11.3	11.9	12.5	13.1	13.7	14.3	14.9
28–32 strokes/min., 1,250 kg·m/min., athletes	12.4	13.1	13.8	14.6	15.3	16.1	16.8	17.6	18.3
28–32 strokes/min., 1,250 kg·m/min., nonathletes	11.6	12.3	13.0	13.7	14.4	15.1	15.8	16.5	17.2
28–32 strokes/min., 1,500 kg·m/min., athletes	14.0	14.9	15.7	16.6	17.4	18.2	19.1	19.9	20.8
28–32 strokes/min., 1,500 kg·m/min., nonathletes	12.9	13.6	14.4	15.2	15.9	16.7	17.5	18.3	19.0
28–32 strokes/min., 1,750 kg·m/min., athletes	15.9	16.8	17.8	18.7	19.7	20.6	21.6	22.5	23.5

Calories Expended by Body Weight

Your Body Weight

77 170	80 176	83 183	86 190	89 196	92 203	95 209	98 216	101 223	104 229	107 236	110 243	113 249	116 256	119 262
18.1	18.8	19.5	20.2	20.9	21.6	22.3	23.0	23.7	24.4	25.1	25.8	26.5	27.2	27.9
5.0	5.2	5.4	5.6	5.8	6.0	6.2	6.3	6.5	6.7	6.9	7.1	7.3	7.5	7.7
17.2	17.9	18.6	19.3	19.9	20.6	21.3	22.0	22.6	23.3	24.0	24.6	25.3	26.0	26.7
24.5	25.5	26.4	27.4	28.3	29.3	30.3	31.2	32.2	33.1	34.1	35.0	36.0	36.9	37.9
17.2	17.9	18.6	19.3	19.9	20.6	21.3	22.0	22.6	23.3	24.0	24.6	25.3	26.0	26.7
18.6	19.4	20.1	20.8	21.5	22.3	23.0	23.7	24.4	25.2	25.9	26.6	27.3	28.1	28.8
16.9	17.5	18.2	18.8	19.5	20.1	20.8	21.5	22.1	22.8	23.4	24.1	24.7	25.4	26.1
13.7	14.2	14.8	15.3	15.8	16.4	16.9	17.4	18.0	18.5	19.0	19.6	20.1	20.6	21.2
20.6	21.4	22.2	23.0	23.8	24.6	25.4	26.2	27.0	27.8	28.6	29.4	30.2	31.0	31.8
14.1	14.6	15.2	15.7	16.3	16.8	17.4	17.9	18.5	19.0	19.6	20.1	20.7	21.2	21.8
16.5	17.1	17.7	18.4	19.0	19.7	20.3	21.0	21.6	22.2	22.9	23.5	24.2	24.8	25.4
15.5	16.1	16.7	17.3	17.9	18.5	19.2	19.8	20.4	21.0	21.6	22.2	22.8	23.4	24.0
19.0	19.8	20.5	21.3	22.0	22.7	23.5	24.2	25.0	25.7	26.5	27.2	27.9	28.7	29.4
17.9	18.6	19.3	20.0	20.7	21.4	22.1	22.8	23.5	24.2	24.9	25.6	26.3	27.0	27.7
21.6	22.5	23.3	24.1	25.0	25.8	26.7	27.5	28.4	29.2	30.0	30.9	31.7	32.6	33.4
19.8	20.6	21.4	22.1	22.9	23.7	24.4	25.2	26.0	26.8	27.5	28.3	29.1	29.8	30.6
24.4	25.4	26.3	27.3	28.3	29.2	30.2	31.1	32.1	33.0	34.0	34.9	35.9	36.8	37.8

Calories Expended by Body Weight

Activity	kg lb	50 110	53 117	56 123	59 130	62 137	65 143	68 150	71 157	74 163
Rowing—Stationary Ergometer										
50 watts, light effort		3.1	3.2	3.4	3.6	3.8	4.0	4.2	4.3	4.5
100 watts, moderate effort		6.1	6.5	6.9	7.2	7.6	8.0	8.3	8.7	9.1
150 watts, vigorous effort		7.4	7.9	8.3	8.8	9.2	9.7	10.1	10.6	11.0
200 watts, very vigorous effort		10.5	11.1	11.8	12.4	13.0	13.7	14.3	14.9	15.5
General		8.3	8.8	9.3	9.8	10.3	10.8	11.3	11.8	12.3
Rugby		8.8	9.3	9.8	10.3	10.9	11.4	11.9	12.4	13.0
Running—General										
5 mph (12 min./mile)		7.0	7.4	7.8	8.3	8.7	9.1	9.5	9.9	10.4
5.2 mph (11.5 min./mile)		7.9	8.3	8.8	9.3	9.8	10.2	10.7	11.2	11.7
6 mph (10 min./mile)		8.8	9.3	9.8	10.3	10.9	11.4	11.9	12.4	13.0
6 mph, carrying 1 lb weights		9.9	10.5	11.1	11.7	12.3	12.9	13.5	14.1	14.6
6 mph, carrying 5 lb weights		10.5	11.1	11.8	12.4	13.0	13.7	14.3	14.9	15.5
6.7 mph (9 min./mile)		9.6	10.2	10.8	11.4	11.9	12.5	13.1	13.7	14.2
7 mph (8.5 min./mile)		10.1	10.7	11.3	11.9	12.5	13.1	13.7	14.3	14.9
7.5 mph (8 min./mile)		10.9	11.6	12.3	12.9	13.6	14.2	14.9	15.5	16.2
8 mph (7.5 min./mile)		11.8	12.5	13.2	13.9	14.6	15.4	16.1	16.8	17.5
8.6 mph (7 min./mile)		12.3	13.0	13.7	14.5	15.2	15.9	16.7	17.4	18.1
8.6 mph, 4% grade, normal stride length		14.2	15.0	15.9	16.7	17.6	18.5	19.3	20.2	21.0
8.6 mph, exaggerated long strides		13.0	13.7	14.5	15.3	16.1	16.8	17.6	18.4	19.2
8.6 mph, exaggerated short, choppy strides		12.5	13.2	14.0	14.7	15.5	16.2	17.0	17.7	18.5
8.6 mph, level grade, normal stride length		11.2	11.9	12.6	13.3	13.9	14.6	15.3	16.0	16.6
9 mph (6.5 min./mile)		13.1	13.9	14.7	15.5	16.3	17.1	17.9	18.6	19.4
10 mph (6 min./mile)		14.0	14.8	15.7	16.5	17.4	18.2	19.0	19.9	20.7
10.9 mph (5.5 min./mile)		15.8	16.7	17.6	18.6	19.5	20.5	21.4	22.4	23.3
Around track, team practice		8.8	9.3	9.8	10.3	10.9	11.4	11.9	12.4	13.0
Backward, 6 mph (10 min./mile)		11.7	12.4	13.1	13.8	14.5	15.2	15.9	16.6	17.3
Cross-country, general, no hills		7.9	8.3	8.8	9.3	9.8	10.2	10.7	11.2	11.7
Cross-country, up and down hills		8.6	9.1	9.6	10.1	10.6	11.1	11.6	12.2	12.7
Downhill, -3% grade, 8.6 mph (7 min./mile)		9.9	10.5	11.1	11.7	12.3	12.9	13.5	14.1	14.6
Downhill, -6% grade, 8.6 mph (7 min./mile)		8.8	9.3	9.9	10.4	10.9	11.4	12.0	12.5	13.0

Calories Expended by Body Weight

Your Body Weight

77 170	80 176	83 183	86 190	89 196	92 203	95 209	98 216	101 223	104 229	107 236	110 243	113 249	116 256	119 262
4.7	4.9	5.1	5.3	5.5	5.6	5.8	6.0	6.2	6.4	6.6	6.7	6.9	7.1	7.3
9.4	9.8	10.2	10.5	10.9	11.3	11.6	12.0	12.4	12.7	13.1	13.5	13.8	14.2	14.6
11.5	11.9	12.3	12.8	13.2	13.7	14.1	14.6	15.0	15.5	15.9	16.4	16.8	17.3	17.7
16.2	16.8	17.4	18.1	18.7	19.3	20.0	20.6	21.2	21.8	22.5	23.1	23.7	24.4	25.0
12.8	13.3	13.8	14.3	14.8	15.3	15.8	16.3	16.8	17.3	17.8	18.3	18.8	19.3	19.8
13.5	14.0	14.5	15.1	15.6	16.1	16.6	17.2	17.7	18.2	18.7	19.3	19.8	20.3	20.8
10.8	11.2	11.6	12.0	12.5	12.9	13.3	13.7	14.1	14.6	15.0	15.4	15.8	16.2	16.7
12.1	12.6	13.1	13.5	14.0	14.5	15.0	15.4	15.9	16.4	16.9	17.3	17.8	18.3	18.7
13.5	14.0	14.5	15.1	15.6	16.1	16.6	17.2	17.7	18.2	18.7	19.3	19.8	20.3	20.8
15.2	15.8	16.4	17.0	17.6	18.2	18.8	19.4	20.0	20.6	21.2	21.8	22.4	23.0	23.6
16.2	16.8	17.4	18.1	18.7	19.3	20.0	20.6	21.2	21.8	22.5	23.1	23.7	24.4	25.0
14.8	15.4	16.0	16.6	17.1	17.7	18.3	18.9	19.4	20.0	20.6	21.2	21.8	22.3	22.9
15.5	16.1	16.7	17.3	17.9	18.5	19.1	19.7	20.3	20.9	21.5	22.1	22.7	23.3	23.9
16.8	17.5	18.2	18.8	19.5	20.1	20.8	21.4	22.1	22.8	23.4	24.1	24.7	25.4	26.0
18.2	18.9	19.6	20.3	21.0	21.7	22.4	23.2	23.9	24.6	25.3	26.0	26.7	27.4	28.1
18.9	19.6	20.3	21.1	21.8	22.5	23.3	24.0	24.7	25.5	26.2	27.0	27.7	28.4	29.2
21.9	22.7	23.6	24.4	25.3	26.1	27.0	27.8	28.7	29.5	30.4	31.2	32.1	32.9	33.8
19.9	20.7	21.5	22.3	23.1	23.8	24.6	25.4	26.2	26.9	27.7	28.5	29.3	30.0	30.8
19.2	20.0	20.7	21.4	22.2	22.9	23.7	24.4	25.2	25.9	26.7	27.4	28.2	28.9	29.7
17.3	18.0	18.7	19.3	20.0	20.7	21.3	22.0	22.7	23.4	24.0	24.7	25.4	26.1	26.7
20.2	21.0	21.8	22.6	23.4	24.2	24.9	25.7	26.5	27.3	28.1	28.9	29.7	30.5	31.2
21.6	22.4	23.2	24.1	24.9	25.8	26.6	27.4	28.3	29.1	30.0	30.8	31.6	32.5	33.3
24.3	25.2	26.1	27.1	28.0	29.0	29.9	30.9	31.8	32.8	33.7	34.7	35.6	36.5	37.5
13.5	14.0	14.5	15.1	15.6	16.1	16.6	17.2	17.7	18.2	18.7	19.3	19.8	20.3	20.8
18.0	18.7	19.4	20.1	20.8	21.5	22.2	22.9	23.6	24.3	25.0	25.7	26.4	27.1	27.8
12.1	12.6	13.1	13.5	14.0	14.5	15.0	15.4	15.9	16.4	16.9	17.3	17.8	18.3	18.7
13.2	13.7	14.2	14.7	15.2	15.7	16.3	16.8	17.3	17.8	18.3	18.8	19.3	19.9	20.4
15.2	15.8	16.4	17.0	17.6	18.2	18.8	19.4	20.0	20.6	21.2	21.8	22.4	23.0	23.6
13.6	14.1	14.6	15.1	15.7	16.2	16.7	17.3	17.8	18.3	18.8	19.4	19.9	20.4	20.9

Calories Expended by Body Weight

Activity	kg lb	50 110	53 117	56 123	59 130	62 137	65 143	68 150	71 157	74 163
Running—General (cont.)										
Downhill, -9% grade, 8.6 mph (7 min./mile)		8.3	8.8	9.3	9.8	10.3	10.8	11.3	11.8	12.3
In place (moderate pace)		7.0	7.4	7.8	8.3	8.7	9.1	9.5	9.9	10.4
Self-selected pace (7–11 min./mile), wearing 1 lb ankle weights		9.0	9.5	10.0	10.6	11.1	11.7	12.2	12.7	13.3
Self-selected pace (7–11 min./mile), wearing hand and ankle weights (2.2–6 lb total)		9.2	9.7	10.3	10.8	11.3	11.9	12.4	13.0	13.5
Self-selected pace (7–11 min./mile), wearing 1–2 lb hand weights		8.9	9.5	10.0	10.5	11.1	11.6	12.1	12.7	13.2
Training, pushing wheelchair, marathon wheeling		7.0	7.4	7.8	8.3	8.7	9.1	9.5	9.9	10.4
Upstairs		13.1	13.9	14.7	15.5	16.3	17.1	17.9	18.6	19.4
Running—In Water										
Deep water (2.5 to 4.0 m depth), no vest, maximal effort		12.1	12.8	13.5	14.3	15.0	15.7	16.4	17.2	17.9
Deep water, wearing flotation device (Wet Vest), maximal effort		10.7	11.4	12.0	12.7	13.3	13.9	14.6	15.2	15.9
Shallow water (1.3 m depth), no vest, maximal effort		15.0	15.9	16.8	17.7	18.6	19.5	20.4	21.3	22.2
Running—Jogging										
General		6.1	6.5	6.9	7.2	7.6	8.0	8.3	8.7	9.1
Jog/Walk combination (jogging component less than 10 min.)		5.3	5.6	5.9	6.2	6.5	6.8	7.1	7.5	7.8
Running—Marathon										
5 h. 02 min. (11:30 min./mile; 140 m/min.)		5.8	6.2	6.5	6.9	7.2	7.6	7.9	8.3	8.6
4 h. 42 min. (10:45 min./mile; 150 m/min.)		6.3	6.7	7.1	7.5	7.9	8.2	8.6	9.0	9.4
4 h. 24 min. (10:05 min./mile; 160 m/min.)		6.9	7.3	7.7	8.1	8.5	8.9	9.3	9.7	10.1
4h. 10min. (10:05 min./mile; 170 m/min.)		7.4	7.8	8.2	8.7	9.1	9.6	10.0	10.5	10.9
3 h. 55 min. (9:00 min./mile; 180 m/min.)		7.9	8.3	8.8	9.3	9.8	10.2	10.7	11.2	11.6

Calories Expended by Body Weight

Your Body Weight

77 170	80 176	83 183	86 190	89 196	92 203	95 209	98 216	101 223	104 229	107 236	110 243	113 249	116 256	119 262
12.8	13.3	13.8	14.3	14.8	15.3	15.8	16.3	16.8	17.3	17.8	18.3	18.8	19.3	19.8
10.8	11.2	11.6	12.0	12.5	12.9	13.3	13.7	14.1	14.6	15.0	15.4	15.8	16.2	16.7
13.8	14.4	14.9	15.4	16.0	16.5	17.0	17.6	18.1	18.7	19.2	19.7	20.3	20.8	21.3
14.1	14.6	15.2	15.7	16.3	16.8	17.4	17.9	18.5	19.0	19.6	20.1	20.7	21.2	21.8
13.7	14.3	14.8	15.4	15.9	16.4	17.0	17.5	18.0	18.6	19.1	19.6	20.2	20.7	21.2
10.8	11.2	11.6	12.0	12.5	12.9	13.3	13.7	14.1	14.6	15.0	15.4	15.8	16.2	16.7
20.2	21.0	21.8	22.6	23.4	24.2	24.9	25.7	26.5	27.3	28.1	28.9	29.7	30.5	31.2
18.6	19.3	20.1	20.8	21.5	22.3	23.0	23.7	24.4	25.2	25.9	26.6	27.3	28.1	28.8
16.5	17.2	17.8	18.5	19.1	19.7	20.4	21.0	21.7	22.3	23.0	23.6	24.2	24.9	25.5
23.1	24.0	24.9	25.8	26.6	27.5	28.4	29.3	30.2	31.1	32.0	32.9	33.8	34.7	35.6
9.4	9.8	10.2	10.5	10.9	11.3	11.6	12.0	12.4	12.7	13.1	13.5	13.8	14.2	14.6
8.1	8.4	8.7	9.0	9.3	9.7	10.0	10.3	10.6	10.9	11.2	11.6	11.9	12.2	12.5
9.0	9.3	9.7	10.0	10.4	10.7	11.1	11.4	11.8	12.1	12.5	12.8	13.2	13.5	13.9
9.8	10.1	10.5	10.9	11.3	11.7	12.1	12.4	12.8	13.2	13.6	14.0	14.3	14.7	15.1
10.6	11.0	11.4	11.8	12.2	12.6	13.0	13.4	13.8	14.3	14.7	15.1	15.5	15.9	16.3
11.3	11.8	12.2	12.7	13.1	13.5	14.0	14.4	14.9	15.3	15.8	16.2	16.6	17.1	17.5
12.1	12.6	13.1	13.5	14.0	14.5	14.9	15.4	15.9	16.4	16.8	17.3	17.8	18.2	18.7

Calories Expended by Body Weight

Your Body Weight

Activity	kg 50 lb 110	53 117	56 123	59 130	62 137	65 143	68 150	71 157	74 163
Running—Marathon (cont.)									
3 h. 43 min. (8:30 min./mile; 190 m/min.)	8.4	8.9	9.4	9.9	10.4	10.9	11.4	11.9	12.4
3 h. 31 min. (8:05 min./mile; 200 m/min.)	8.9	9.4	10.0	10.5	11.0	11.6	12.1	12.6	13.2
3 h. 21 min. (7:40 min./mile; 210 m/min.)	9.4	10.0	10.5	11.1	11.7	12.2	12.8	13.3	13.9
3 h. 12 min. (7:20 min./mile; 220 m/min.)	9.9	10.5	11.1	11.7	12.3	12.9	13.5	14.1	14.7
3 h. 04 min. (7:00 min./mile; 230 m/min.)	10.4	11.0	11.7	12.3	12.9	13.5	14.2	14.8	15.4
2 h. 56 min. (6:45 min./mile; 240 m/min.)	10.9	11.6	12.2	12.9	13.6	14.2	14.9	15.5	16.2
2 h. 49 min. (6:27 min./mile; 250 m/min.)	11.4	12.1	12.8	13.5	14.2	14.9	15.6	16.2	16.9
2 h. 43 min. (6:12 min./mile; 260 m/min.)	12.0	12.7	13.4	14.1	14.8	15.5	16.3	17.0	17.7
2 h. 37 min. (6:00 min./mile; 270 m/min.)	12.5	13.2	14.0	14.7	15.5	16.2	16.9	17.7	18.4
2 h. 31 min. (5:45 min./mile; 280 m/min.)	13.0	13.7	14.5	15.3	16.1	16.9	17.6	18.4	19.2
2 h. 26 min. (5:34 min./mile; 290 m/min.)	13.5	14.3	15.1	15.9	16.7	17.5	18.3	19.1	20.0
2 h. 21 min. (5:23 min./mile; 300 m/min.)	14.0	14.8	15.7	16.5	17.4	18.2	19.0	19.9	20.7
2 h. 16 min. (5:12 min./mile; 310 m/min.)	14.5	15.4	16.2	17.1	18.0	18.9	19.7	20.6	21.5
2 h. 12 min. (5:03 min./mile; 320 m/min.)	15.0	15.9	16.8	17.7	18.6	19.5	20.4	21.3	22.2
2 h. 08 min. (4:54 min./mile; 330 m/min.)	15.5	16.5	17.4	18.3	19.3	20.2	21.1	22.0	23.0
Sailing									
Boat and board sailing, general	3.4	3.6	3.8	4.0	4.2	4.4	4.6	4.8	5.1
Competition	4.4	4.6	4.9	5.2	5.4	5.7	6.0	6.2	6.5
Putting on and removing tarp	2.6	2.8	2.9	3.1	3.3	3.4	3.6	3.7	3.9
Scraping and painting sailboat or powerboat	3.9	4.2	4.4	4.6	4.9	5.1	5.4	5.6	5.8

Calories Expended by Body Weight

Your Body Weight

77 170	80 176	83 183	86 190	89 196	92 203	95 209	98 216	101 223	104 229	107 236	110 243	113 249	116 256	119 262
12.9	13.4	13.9	14.4	14.9	15.4	15.9	16.4	16.9	17.4	17.9	18.4	18.9	19.4	20.0
13.7	14.2	14.8	15.3	15.8	16.4	16.9	17.4	18.0	18.5	19.0	19.6	20.1	20.6	21.2
14.5	15.0	15.6	16.2	16.7	17.3	17.9	18.4	19.0	19.5	20.1	20.7	21.2	21.8	22.4
15.3	15.9	16.5	17.1	17.6	18.2	18.8	19.4	20.0	20.6	21.2	21.8	22.4	23.0	23.6
16.0	16.7	17.3	17.9	18.5	19.2	19.8	20.4	21.1	21.7	22.3	22.9	23.6	24.2	24.8
16.8	17.5	18.1	18.8	19.5	20.1	20.8	21.4	22.1	22.7	23.4	24.0	24.7	25.4	26.0
17.6	18.3	19.0	19.7	20.4	21.0	21.7	22.4	23.1	23.8	24.5	25.2	25.8	26.5	27.2
18.4	19.1	19.8	20.6	21.3	22.0	22.7	23.4	24.1	24.9	25.6	26.3	27.0	27.7	28.4
19.2	19.9	20.7	21.4	22.2	22.9	23.7	24.4	25.2	25.9	26.7	27.4	28.2	28.9	29.7
20.0	20.7	21.5	22.3	23.1	23.9	24.6	25.4	26.2	27.0	27.8	28.5	29.3	30.1	30.9
20.8	21.6	22.4	23.2	24.0	24.8	25.6	26.4	27.2	28.0	28.9	29.7	30.5	31.3	32.1
21.6	22.4	23.2	24.1	24.9	25.7	26.6	27.4	28.3	29.1	29.9	30.8	31.6	32.5	33.3
22.3	23.2	24.1	24.9	25.8	26.7	27.6	28.4	29.3	30.2	31.0	31.9	32.8	33.7	34.5
23.1	24.0	24.9	25.8	26.7	27.6	28.5	29.4	30.3	31.2	32.1	33.0	33.9	34.8	35.7
23.9	24.8	25.8	26.7	27.6	28.6	29.5	30.4	31.4	32.3	33.2	34.2	35.1	36.0	36.9

5.3	5.5	5.7	5.9	6.1	6.3	6.5	6.7	6.9	7.1	7.3	7.5	7.7	7.9	8.1
6.7	7.0	7.3	7.5	7.8	8.1	8.3	8.6	8.8	9.1	9.4	9.6	9.9	10.2	10.4
4.0	4.2	4.4	4.5	4.7	4.8	5.0	5.1	5.3	5.5	5.6	5.8	5.9	6.1	6.2
6.1	6.3	6.5	6.8	7.0	7.2	7.5	7.7	8.0	8.2	8.4	8.7	8.9	9.1	9.4

Calories Expended by Body Weight

Activity	kg	50	53	56	59	62	65	68	71	74
	lb	110	117	123	130	137	143	150	157	163
Sunfish/Laser/Hobbie Cat, keel boats, ocean sailing, yachting		2.6	2.8	2.9	3.1	3.3	3.4	3.6	3.7	3.9
Washing and waxing hull of sailboat or powerboat		3.9	4.2	4.4	4.6	4.9	5.1	5.4	5.6	5.8
Sanding Floors (Power Sander)		3.9	4.2	4.4	4.6	4.9	5.1	5.4	5.6	5.8
Scrubbing Floors (Hands and Knees)		4.8	5.1	5.4	5.7	6.0	6.3	6.5	6.8	7.1
Scuba Diving										
General, recreational		6.6	7.0	7.4	7.7	8.1	8.5	8.9	9.3	9.7
Underwater finning, maximal effort		10.6	11.2	11.9	12.5	13.1	13.8	14.4	15.0	15.7
Security Guard										
Laser-weapon-combat field maneuvers		3.9	4.2	4.4	4.6	4.9	5.1	5.4	5.6	5.8
Routine daily work over 12 hr. duration		1.8	1.9	2.0	2.1	2.2	2.3	2.4	2.5	2.6
Sexual Activity										
Passive, light effort (kissing, hugging)		1.1	1.2	1.2	1.3	1.4	1.4	1.5	1.6	1.6
Moderate effort (kissing, hugging, petting-fondling)		1.3	1.4	1.5	1.6	1.6	1.7	1.8	1.9	2.0
Vigorous effort (intercourse)		1.5	1.6	1.7	1.8	1.8	1.9	2.0	2.1	2.2
Shoe Repair (General)		2.2	2.3	2.5	2.6	2.7	2.8	3.0	3.1	3.2
Shopping (without Cart)		2.2	2.3	2.5	2.6	2.7	2.8	3.0	3.1	3.2
Shoveling										
Digging ditches		7.4	7.9	8.3	8.8	9.2	9.7	10.1	10.6	11.0
Light (less than 10 lb/min.)		5.3	5.6	5.9	6.2	6.5	6.8	7.1	7.5	7.8
Moderate (10-15 lb/min.)		6.1	6.5	6.9	7.2	7.6	8.0	8.3	8.7	9.1
Heavy (more than 16 lb/min.)		7.9	8.3	8.8	9.3	9.8	10.2	10.7	11.2	11.7
Shoveling grain		4.8	5.1	5.4	5.7	6.0	6.3	6.5	6.8	7.1
Shoveling snow by hand		5.3	5.6	5.9	6.2	6.5	6.8	7.1	7.5	7.8
Spreading dirt with a shovel		4.4	4.6	4.9	5.2	5.4	5.7	6.0	6.2	6.5

Calories Expended by Body Weight

Your Body Weight

77 170	80 176	83 183	86 190	89 196	92 203	95 209	98 216	101 223	104 229	107 236	110 243	113 249	116 256	119 262
4.0	4.2	4.4	4.5	4.7	4.8	5.0	5.1	5.3	5.5	5.6	5.8	5.9	6.1	6.2
6.1	6.3	6.5	6.8	7.0	7.2	7.5	7.7	8.0	8.2	8.4	8.7	8.9	9.1	9.4
6.1	6.3	6.5	6.8	7.0	7.2	7.5	7.7	8.0	8.2	8.4	8.7	8.9	9.1	9.4
7.4	7.7	8.0	8.3	8.6	8.9	9.1	9.4	9.7	10.0	10.3	10.6	10.9	11.2	11.5
10.1	10.5	10.9	11.3	11.7	12.1	12.5	12.9	13.3	13.7	14.0	14.4	14.8	15.2	15.6
16.3	16.9	17.6	18.2	18.8	19.5	20.1	20.8	21.4	22.0	22.7	23.3	23.9	24.6	25.2
6.1	6.3	6.5	6.8	7.0	7.2	7.5	7.7	8.0	8.2	8.4	8.7	8.9	9.1	9.4
2.7	2.8	2.9	3.0	3.1	3.2	3.3	3.4	3.5	3.6	3.7	3.9	4.0	4.1	4.2
1.7	1.8	1.8	1.9	1.9	2.0	2.1	2.1	2.2	2.3	2.3	2.4	2.5	2.5	2.6
2.0	2.1	2.2	2.3	2.4	2.4	2.5	2.6	2.7	2.8	2.8	2.9	3.0	3.1	3.2
2.3	2.4	2.5	2.6	2.6	2.7	2.8	2.9	3.0	3.1	3.2	3.3	3.4	3.5	3.5
3.4	3.5	3.6	3.8	3.9	4.0	4.2	4.3	4.4	4.6	4.7	4.8	4.9	5.1	5.2
3.4	3.5	3.6	3.8	3.9	4.0	4.2	4.3	4.4	4.6	4.7	4.8	4.9	5.1	5.2
11.5	11.9	12.3	12.8	13.2	13.7	14.1	14.6	15.0	15.5	15.9	16.4	16.8	17.3	17.7
8.1	8.4	8.7	9.0	9.3	9.7	10.0	10.3	10.6	10.9	11.2	11.6	11.9	12.2	12.5
9.4	9.8	10.2	10.5	10.9	11.3	11.6	12.0	12.4	12.7	13.1	13.5	13.8	14.2	14.6
12.1	12.6	13.1	13.5	14.0	14.5	15.0	15.4	15.9	16.4	16.9	17.3	17.8	18.3	18.7
7.4	7.7	8.0	8.3	8.6	8.9	9.1	9.4	9.7	10.0	10.3	10.6	10.9	11.2	11.5
8.1	8.4	8.7	9.0	9.3	9.7	10.0	10.3	10.6	10.9	11.2	11.6	11.9	12.2	12.5
6.7	7.0	7.3	7.5	7.8	8.1	8.3	8.6	8.8	9.1	9.4	9.6	9.9	10.2	10.4

Calories Expended by Body Weight

Activity	kg lb	50 110	53 117	56 123	59 130	62 137	65 143	68 150	71 157	74 163
Showering *(Toweling Off, Standing)*		3.5	3.7	3.9	4.1	4.3	4.6	4.8	5.0	5.2
Shuffleboard—Lawn Bowling		2.6	2.8	2.9	3.1	3.3	3.4	3.6	3.7	3.9
Sitting General—class, note-taking, discussion		1.6	1.7	1.8	1.9	2.0	2.0	2.1	2.2	2.3
Grooming (washing, shaving, brushing teeth, putting on makeup)		2.2	2.3	2.5	2.6	2.7	2.8	3.0	3.1	3.2
Knitting, sewing, gift wrapping		1.3	1.4	1.5	1.5	1.6	1.7	1.8	1.9	1.9
Light office work, general (lab work, light use of hand tools, light assembly/repair)		1.3	1.4	1.5	1.5	1.6	1.7	1.8	1.9	1.9
Meetings, general, or with talking involved		1.3	1.4	1.5	1.5	1.6	1.7	1.8	1.9	1.9
Moderate (heavy levers, riding mower/forklift, crane operation)		2.2	2.3	2.5	2.6	2.7	2.8	3.0	3.1	3.2
Playing cards, board games, doing homework		1.3	1.4	1.5	1.5	1.6	1.7	1.8	1.9	1.9
Playing with children—light		2.2	2.3	2.5	2.6	2.7	2.8	3.0	3.1	3.2
Reading, surfing Internet		1.0	1.1	1.2	1.2	1.3	1.4	1.4	1.5	1.5
Sitting quietly (riding in car, listening to lecture, music, watching TV)		0.9	1.0	1.0	1.1	1.2	1.2	1.3	1.3	1.4
Studying, general, including reading and/or writing		1.6	1.7	1.8	1.9	2.0	2.0	2.1	2.2	2.3
Talking		1.3	1.4	1.5	1.5	1.6	1.7	1.8	1.9	1.9
Toilet		1.0	1.0	1.1	1.2	1.2	1.3	1.3	1.4	1.5
Writing, desk work, computer work		1.6	1.7	1.8	1.9	2.0	2.0	2.1	2.2	2.3
Skateboarding		4.4	4.6	4.9	5.2	5.4	5.7	6.0	6.2	6.5
Skiing—Cross Country (Nordic) 2.5 mph, light effort, ski walking		6.4	6.8	7.2	7.5	7.9	8.3	8.7	9.1	9.5
4.0 to 4.9 mph, moderate speed and effort, general		7.4	7.8	8.2	8.7	9.1	9.6	10.0	10.4	10.9
5.0 to 7.9 mph, vigorous effort		8.1	8.6	9.1	9.6	10.1	10.5	11.0	11.5	12.0

Calories Expended by Body Weight

Your Body Weight

77 170	80 176	83 183	86 190	89 196	92 203	95 209	98 216	101 223	104 229	107 236	110 243	113 249	116 256	119 262
5.4	5.6	5.8	6.0	6.2	6.4	6.7	6.9	7.1	7.3	7.5	7.7	7.9	8.1	8.3
4.0	4.2	4.4	4.5	4.7	4.8	5.0	5.1	5.3	5.5	5.6	5.8	5.9	6.1	6.2
2.4	2.5	2.6	2.7	2.8	2.9	3.0	3.1	3.2	3.3	3.4	3.5	3.6	3.7	3.7
3.4	3.5	3.6	3.8	3.9	4.0	4.2	4.3	4.4	4.6	4.7	4.8	4.9	5.1	5.2
2.0	2.1	2.2	2.3	2.3	2.4	2.5	2.6	2.7	2.7	2.8	2.9	3.0	3.0	3.1
2.0	2.1	2.2	2.3	2.3	2.4	2.5	2.6	2.7	2.7	2.8	2.9	3.0	3.0	3.1
2.0	2.1	2.2	2.3	2.3	2.4	2.5	2.6	2.7	2.7	2.8	2.9	3.0	3.0	3.1
3.4	3.5	3.6	3.8	3.9	4.0	4.2	4.3	4.4	4.6	4.7	4.8	4.9	5.1	5.2
2.0	2.1	2.2	2.3	2.3	2.4	2.5	2.6	2.7	2.7	2.8	2.9	3.0	3.0	3.1
3.4	3.5	3.6	3.8	3.9	4.0	4.2	4.3	4.4	4.6	4.7	4.8	4.9	5.1	5.2
1.6	1.7	1.7	1.8	1.9	1.9	2.0	2.0	2.1	2.2	2.2	2.3	2.4	2.4	2.5
1.4	1.5	1.5	1.6	1.7	1.7	1.8	1.8	1.9	1.9	2.0	2.0	2.1	2.2	2.2
2.4	2.5	2.6	2.7	2.8	2.9	3.0	3.1	3.2	3.3	3.4	3.5	3.6	3.7	3.7
2.0	2.1	2.2	2.3	2.3	2.4	2.5	2.6	2.7	2.7	2.8	2.9	3.0	3.0	3.1
1.5	1.6	1.6	1.7	1.7	1.8	1.9	1.9	2.0	2.0	2.1	2.2	2.2	2.3	2.3
2.4	2.5	2.6	2.7	2.8	2.9	3.0	3.1	3.2	3.3	3.4	3.5	3.6	3.7	3.7
6.7	7.0	7.3	7.5	7.8	8.1	8.3	8.6	8.8	9.1	9.4	9.6	9.9	10.2	10.4
9.8	10.2	10.6	11.0	11.4	11.8	12.1	12.5	12.9	13.3	13.7	14.1	14.4	14.8	15.2
11.3	11.8	12.2	12.6	13.1	13.5	14.0	14.4	14.8	15.3	15.7	16.2	16.6	17.1	17.5
12.5	13.0	13.5	14.0	14.4	14.9	15.4	15.9	16.4	16.9	17.4	17.8	18.3	18.8	19.3

Calories Expended by Body Weight

					Your Body Weight				
Activity	**kg 50** **lb 110**	**53** **117**	**56** **123**	**59** **130**	**62** **137**	**65** **143**	**68** **150**	**71** **157**	**74** **163**
Skiing—Cross Country (Nordic) (cont.)									
8.9 mph, double pole, traditional skis	10.3	10.9	11.5	12.1	12.7	13.4	14.0	14.6	15.2
8.9 mph, double pole, skating skis	9.1	9.6	10.2	10.7	11.3	11.8	12.4	12.9	13.5
8.9 mph, kick, double pole	8.7	9.2	9.8	10.3	10.8	11.3	11.9	12.4	12.9
8.9 mph, kick, diagonal stride	12.0	12.7	13.4	14.2	14.9	15.6	16.3	17.0	17.8
8.9 mph, marathon skate	10.2	10.9	11.5	12.1	12.7	13.3	13.9	14.5	15.2
8.9 mph, V-Skate skate	9.8	10.4	11.0	11.6	12.2	12.7	13.3	13.9	14.5
Hard snow, uphill (5% grade), maximal effort	19.3	20.4	21.6	22.7	23.9	25.0	26.2	27.3	28.5
Hard snow, uphill, recreational	14.4	15.3	16.2	17.0	17.9	18.8	19.6	20.5	21.4
Skiing—Downhill (Alpine)									
Light effort	4.9	5.2	5.5	5.8	6.1	6.4	6.7	7.0	7.3
Moderate effort, general	5.5	5.8	6.2	6.5	6.8	7.2	7.5	7.8	8.2
Vigorous effort, racing	7.0	7.4	7.8	8.3	8.7	9.1	9.5	9.9	10.4
Skiing—Machines									
Fitness Master model LT-35, 76% of max heart rate (145 beats/min.)	7.5	7.9	8.4	8.8	9.3	9.7	10.2	10.6	11.1
Fitness Master model LT-35, 82% of max heart rate (155 beats/min.)	8.4	8.9	9.4	9.9	10.4	10.9	11.4	11.9	12.4
Fitness Master model LT-35, 87% of max heart rate (165 beats/min.)	9.2	9.7	10.3	10.8	11.4	11.9	12.5	13.0	13.6
Fitness Master model LT-35, maximal effort	11.9	12.6	13.3	14.0	14.8	15.5	16.2	16.9	17.6
NordicSport downhill ski ergometer (86 turns/min.), men	8.3	8.8	9.3	9.8	10.3	10.8	11.3	11.8	12.3
NordicSport downhill ski ergometer (86 turns/min.), women	7.3	7.7	8.2	8.6	9.1	9.5	9.9	10.4	10.8
NordicTrak FITONE, self-selected pace	8.6	9.1	9.6	10.1	10.6	11.1	11.6	12.2	12.7
NordicTrak model 530, 76% of max heart rate (145 beats/min.)	8.2	8.7	9.2	9.7	10.2	10.7	11.2	11.7	12.2

Calories Expended by Body Weight

Your Body Weight

77 170	80 176	83 183	86 190	89 196	92 203	95 209	98 216	101 223	104 229	107 236	110 243	113 249	116 256	119 262
15.8	16.4	17.1	17.7	18.3	18.9	19.5	20.1	20.8	21.4	22.0	22.6	23.2	23.8	24.4
14.0	14.6	15.1	15.7	16.2	16.7	17.3	17.8	18.4	18.9	19.5	20.0	20.6	21.1	21.7
13.4	14.0	14.5	15.0	15.5	16.1	16.6	17.1	17.6	18.1	18.7	19.2	19.7	20.2	20.8
18.5	19.2	19.9	20.6	21.4	22.1	22.8	23.5	24.2	25.0	25.7	26.4	27.1	27.8	28.6
15.8	16.4	17.0	17.6	18.2	18.9	19.5	20.1	20.7	21.3	21.9	22.5	23.2	23.8	24.4
15.1	15.7	16.3	16.9	17.4	18.0	18.6	19.2	19.8	20.4	21.0	21.6	22.1	22.7	23.3
29.6	30.8	32.0	33.1	34.3	35.4	36.6	37.7	38.9	40.0	41.2	42.4	43.5	44.7	45.8
22.2	23.1	24.0	24.8	25.7	26.6	27.4	28.3	29.2	30.0	30.9	31.8	32.6	33.5	34.4
7.5	7.8	8.1	8.4	8.7	9.0	9.3	9.6	9.9	10.2	10.5	10.8	11.1	11.4	11.7
8.5	8.8	9.2	9.5	9.8	10.1	10.5	10.8	11.1	11.5	11.8	12.1	12.5	12.8	13.1
10.8	11.2	11.6	12.0	12.5	12.9	13.3	13.7	14.1	14.6	15.0	15.4	15.8	16.2	16.7
11.5	12.0	12.4	12.9	13.3	13.7	14.2	14.6	15.1	15.5	16.0	16.4	16.9	17.3	17.8
12.9	13.4	13.9	14.4	14.9	15.4	15.9	16.4	16.9	17.4	17.9	18.4	18.9	19.4	19.9
14.1	14.7	15.2	15.8	16.3	16.9	17.4	18.0	18.5	19.1	19.6	20.2	20.7	21.3	21.8
18.3	19.0	19.8	20.5	21.2	21.9	22.6	23.3	24.0	24.8	25.5	26.2	26.9	27.6	28.3
12.8	13.3	13.8	14.3	14.8	15.3	15.8	16.3	16.8	17.3	17.8	18.3	18.8	19.3	19.8
11.2	11.7	12.1	12.6	13.0	13.4	13.9	14.3	14.7	15.2	15.6	16.1	16.5	16.9	17.4
13.2	13.7	14.2	14.7	15.2	15.7	16.3	16.8	17.3	17.8	18.3	18.8	19.3	19.9	20.4
12.7	13.2	13.7	14.1	14.6	15.1	15.6	16.1	16.6	17.1	17.6	18.1	18.6	19.1	19.6

		Calories Expended by Body Weight								
					Your Body Weight					
Activity	**kg** **lb**	**50** **110**	**53** **117**	**56** **123**	**59** **130**	**62** **137**	**65** **143**	**68** **150**	**71** **157**	**74** **163**
Skiing—Machines (cont.)										
NordicTrack model 530, 82% of max heart rate (155 beats/min.)		9.0	9.6	10.1	10.6	11.2	11.7	12.3	12.8	13.4
NordicTrack model 530, 87% of max heart rate (165 beats/min.)		10.0	10.6	11.2	11.8	12.4	13.0	13.6	14.2	14.8
NordicTrack model 530, maximal effort		13.0	13.8	14.6	15.4	16.2	16.9	17.7	18.5	19.3
NordicTrack PowerPoles (level, 4.3 mph)		6.0	6.4	6.7	7.1	7.4	7.8	8.2	8.5	8.9
NordicTrack type, general		8.3	8.8	9.3	9.8	10.3	10.8	11.3	11.8	12.3
Skiing—Water										
Competition, slalom		6.4	6.8	7.2	7.5	7.9	8.3	8.7	9.1	9.5
Recreational, 2 skis		5.3	5.6	5.9	6.2	6.5	6.8	7.1	7.5	7.8
Skin Diving										
Frogman		10.6	11.3	11.9	12.5	13.2	13.8	14.4	15.1	15.7
General		6.3	6.7	7.1	7.4	7.8	8.2	8.6	8.9	9.3
Moderate		10.9	11.6	12.3	12.9	13.6	14.2	14.9	15.5	16.2
Vigorous		14.0	14.8	15.7	16.5	17.4	18.2	19.0	19.9	20.7
Sky Diving		3.1	3.2	3.4	3.6	3.8	4.0	4.2	4.3	4.5
Sledding										
Sledding (bobsledding), recreational		6.1	6.5	6.9	7.2	7.6	8.0	8.3	8.7	9.1
Tobogganing		6.5	6.9	7.3	7.6	8.0	8.4	8.8	9.2	9.6
Sleeping		0.9	0.9	1.0	1.0	1.1	1.1	1.2	1.2	1.3
Slideboard Exercise										
66 in. wide polyethylene slideboard performed to 10 min. routine at 30 slides/min.		7.0	7.4	7.8	8.3	8.7	9.1	9.5	9.9	10.4
66 in. wide polyethylene slideboard performed to 10 min. routine at 40 slides/min.		7.7	8.2	8.7	9.1	9.6	10.0	10.5	11.0	11.4

Calories Expended by Body Weight

						Your Body Weight									
77	**80**	**83**	**86**	**89**	**92**	**95**	**98**	**101**	**104**	**107**	**110**	**113**	**116**	**119**
170	**176**	**183**	**190**	**196**	**203**	**209**	**216**	**223**	**229**	**236**	**243**	**249**	**256**	**262**

13.9	14.4	15.0	15.5	16.1	16.6	17.1	17.7	18.2	18.8	19.3	19.8	20.4	20.9	21.5
15.4	16.0	16.6	17.2	17.8	18.4	19.0	19.6	20.1	20.7	21.3	21.9	22.5	23.1	23.7
20.1	20.8	21.6	22.4	23.2	24.0	24.8	25.5	26.3	27.1	27.9	28.7	29.4	30.2	31.0
9.2	9.6	10.0	10.3	10.7	11.0	11.4	11.8	12.1	12.5	12.8	13.2	13.6	13.9	14.3
12.8	13.3	13.8	14.3	14.8	15.3	15.8	16.3	16.8	17.3	17.8	18.3	18.8	19.3	19.8
9.8	10.2	10.6	11.0	11.4	11.8	12.1	12.5	12.9	13.3	13.7	14.1	14.4	14.8	15.2
8.1	8.4	8.7	9.0	9.3	9.7	10.0	10.3	10.6	10.9	11.2	11.6	11.9	12.2	12.5
16.3	17.0	17.6	18.3	18.9	19.5	20.2	20.8	21.4	22.1	22.7	23.4	24.0	24.6	25.3
9.7	10.1	10.5	10.8	11.2	11.6	12.0	12.3	12.7	13.1	13.5	13.9	14.2	14.6	15.0
16.8	17.5	18.2	18.8	19.5	20.1	20.8	21.4	22.1	22.8	23.4	24.1	24.7	25.4	26.0
21.6	22.4	23.2	24.1	24.9	25.8	26.6	27.4	28.3	29.1	30.0	30.8	31.6	32.5	33.3
4.7	4.9	5.1	5.3	5.5	5.6	5.8	6.0	6.2	6.4	6.6	6.7	6.9	7.1	7.3
9.4	9.8	10.2	10.5	10.9	11.3	11.6	12.0	12.4	12.7	13.1	13.5	13.8	14.2	14.6
10.0	10.4	10.7	11.1	11.5	11.9	12.3	12.7	13.1	13.5	13.9	14.2	14.6	15.0	15.4
1.3	1.4	1.5	1.5	1.6	1.6	1.7	1.7	1.8	1.8	1.9	1.9	2.0	2.0	2.1
10.8	11.2	11.6	12.0	12.5	12.9	13.3	13.7	14.1	14.6	15.0	15.4	15.8	16.2	16.7
11.9	12.4	12.8	13.3	13.8	14.2	14.7	15.1	15.6	16.1	16.5	17.0	17.5	17.9	18.4

Calories Expended by Body Weight

Activity		kg 50 lb 110	53 117	56 123	59 130	62 137	65 143	68 150	71 157	74 163
Your Body Weight										

Headers: **Calories Expended by Body Weight** / Your Body Weight

Activity	kg 50 / lb 110	53 / 117	56 / 123	59 / 130	62 / 137	65 / 143	68 / 150	71 / 157	74 / 163
Slideboard Exercise (cont.)									
66 in. wide polyethylene slideboard, performed to 10 min. routine at 40 slides/min., wearing 7.5 lb ankle weights	10.1	10.7	11.3	11.9	12.5	13.1	13.7	14.3	14.9
Slimnastics Exercise (Structured Class Format)	5.3	5.6	5.9	6.2	6.5	6.8	7.1	7.5	7.8
Snorkeling (Pleasure, Not Vigorous)	4.5	4.7	5.0	5.3	5.5	5.8	6.1	6.3	6.6
Snow Blower (Riding)	2.6	2.8	2.9	3.1	3.3	3.4	3.6	3.7	3.9
Snowmobiling	3.1	3.2	3.4	3.6	3.8	4.0	4.2	4.3	4.5
Snowshoeing									
Hiking, open fields, trails	7.0	7.4	7.8	8.3	8.7	9.1	9.5	9.9	10.4
Jogging, moving fast with lightweight snowshoes	12.7	13.4	14.2	15.0	15.7	16.5	17.3	18.0	18.8
Soccer									
Casual, general	6.1	6.5	6.9	7.2	7.6	8.0	8.3	8.7	9.1
Competition	8.8	9.3	9.8	10.3	10.9	11.4	11.9	12.4	13.0
Softball									
Fast or slow pitch, general	4.4	4.6	4.9	5.2	5.4	5.7	6.0	6.2	6.5
Infield/outfield	5.0	5.3	5.6	5.9	6.2	6.5	6.8	7.1	7.4
Officiating	3.5	3.7	3.9	4.1	4.3	4.6	4.8	5.0	5.2
Pitching	5.3	5.6	5.9	6.2	6.5	6.8	7.1	7.5	7.8
Squash	10.5	11.1	11.8	12.4	13.0	13.7	14.3	14.9	15.5
Stair Climbing—General									
Stair-treadmill ergometer, general	5.3	5.6	5.9	6.2	6.5	6.8	7.1	7.5	7.8
With crutches, 16 steps/min., 7.5 in. bench	3.6	3.8	4.0	4.2	4.5	4.7	4.9	5.1	5.3
With crutches, 24 steps/min., 7.5 in. bench	4.8	5.1	5.4	5.7	6.0	6.3	6.6	6.8	7.1

Calories Expended by Body Weight

Your Body Weight

77 170	80 176	83 183	86 190	89 196	92 203	95 209	98 216	101 223	104 229	107 236	110 243	113 249	116 256	119 262
15.5	16.1	16.7	17.3	17.9	18.5	19.1	19.7	20.3	20.9	21.6	22.2	22.8	23.4	24.0
8.1	8.4	8.7	9.0	9.3	9.7	10.0	10.3	10.6	10.9	11.2	11.6	11.9	12.2	12.5
6.9	7.1	7.4	7.7	7.9	8.2	8.5	8.7	9.0	9.3	9.5	9.8	10.1	10.4	10.6
4.0	4.2	4.4	4.5	4.7	4.8	5.0	5.1	5.3	5.5	5.6	5.8	5.9	6.1	6.2
4.7	4.9	5.1	5.3	5.5	5.6	5.8	6.0	6.2	6.4	6.6	6.7	6.9	7.1	7.3
10.8	11.2	11.6	12.0	12.5	12.9	13.3	13.7	14.1	14.6	15.0	15.4	15.8	16.2	16.7
19.5	20.3	21.1	21.8	22.6	23.3	24.1	24.9	25.6	26.4	27.2	27.9	28.7	29.4	30.2
9.4	9.8	10.2	10.5	10.9	11.3	11.6	12.0	12.4	12.7	13.1	13.5	13.8	14.2	14.6
13.5	14.0	14.5	15.1	15.6	16.1	16.6	17.2	17.7	18.2	18.7	19.3	19.8	20.3	20.8
6.7	7.0	7.3	7.5	7.8	8.1	8.3	8.6	8.8	9.1	9.4	9.6	9.9	10.2	10.4
7.7	8.0	8.3	8.6	8.9	9.2	9.5	9.8	10.1	10.4	10.7	11.0	11.3	11.6	11.9
5.4	5.6	5.8	6.0	6.2	6.4	6.7	6.9	7.1	7.3	7.5	7.7	7.9	8.1	8.3
8.1	8.4	8.7	9.0	9.3	9.7	10.0	10.3	10.6	10.9	11.2	11.6	11.9	12.2	12.5
16.2	16.8	17.4	18.1	18.7	19.3	20.0	20.6	21.2	21.8	22.5	23.1	23.7	24.4	25.0
8.1	8.4	8.7	9.0	9.3	9.7	10.0	10.3	10.6	10.9	11.2	11.6	11.9	12.2	12.5
5.5	5.8	6.0	6.2	6.4	6.6	6.8	7.0	7.3	7.5	7.7	7.9	8.1	8.3	8.6
7.4	7.7	8.0	8.3	8.6	8.9	9.2	9.4	9.7	10.0	10.3	10.6	10.9	11.2	11.5

Calories Expended by Body Weight

Activity	kg lb	50 110	53 117	56 123	59 130	62 137	65 143	68 150	71 157	74 163
Stair Climbing—LifeStep										
78% max heart rate, men		8.6	9.1	9.7	10.2	10.7	11.2	11.7	12.3	12.8
78% max heart rate, women		6.3	6.7	7.0	7.4	7.8	8.2	8.5	8.9	9.3
Stair Climbing—Precor Professional Low-Impact Climber										
Level 1 (low): 8 in. step		3.5	3.7	3.9	4.1	4.3	4.5	4.7	4.9	5.1
Level 1 (low): 12 in. step		3.8	4.1	4.3	4.5	4.8	5.0	5.2	5.5	5.7
Level 2 (medium): 8 in. step		3.9	4.1	4.3	4.6	4.8	5.0	5.3	5.5	5.7
Level 3 (medium): 8 in. step		4.1	4.3	4.5	4.8	5.0	5.3	5.5	5.8	6.0
Level 3 (medium): 12 in. step		4.3	4.5	4.8	5.0	5.3	5.5	5.8	6.0	6.3
Stair Climbing—StairMaster 4000										
24 steps/min.		3.5	3.7	3.9	4.1	4.3	4.6	4.8	5.0	5.2
26 steps/min.		3.5	3.7	3.9	4.1	4.3	4.6	4.8	5.0	5.2
30 steps/min.		6.1	6.5	6.9	7.2	7.6	8.0	8.3	8.7	9.1
30 steps/min., holding on		3.5	3.7	3.9	4.1	4.3	4.6	4.8	5.0	5.2
36 steps/min.		8.8	9.3	9.8	10.3	10.9	11.4	11.9	12.4	13.0
36 steps/min., holding on		6.1	6.5	6.9	7.2	7.6	8.0	8.3	8.7	9.1
40 steps/min.		6.1	6.5	6.9	7.2	7.6	8.0	8.3	8.7	9.1
46–48 steps/min.		8.8	9.3	9.8	10.3	10.9	11.4	11.9	12.4	13.0
Stair Climbing—Stairmaster 4000PT										
Rate = 5, 60 steps/min., no holding on		1.8	1.9	2.0	2.1	2.2	2.3	2.4	2.5	2.6
Rate = 7, 77 steps/min., no holding on		2.2	2.3	2.4	2.6	2.7	2.8	2.9	3.1	3.2
Rate = 9, 95 steps/min., no holding on		2.6	2.7	2.9	3.0	3.2	3.3	3.5	3.6	3.8
Rate = 11, 112 steps/min., no holding on		3.0	3.2	3.3	3.5	3.7	3.9	4.1	4.2	4.4
Stairclimbing—Versa Climber										
65% of max heart rate		4.9	5.2	5.5	5.8	6.1	6.4	6.7	7.0	7.3
80% of max heart rate		7.1	7.5	7.9	8.3	8.7	9.2	9.6	10.0	10.4
Maximal effort		7.7	8.1	8.6	9.1	9.5	10.0	10.4	10.9	11.4
Standing										
Drawing (writing), casino gambling		1.8	1.9	2.0	2.1	2.2	2.3	2.4	2.5	2.6
Getting ready for bed		2.2	2.3	2.5	2.6	2.7	2.8	3.0	3.1	3.2

Calories Expended by Body Weight

Your Body Weight														
77 **170**	**80** **176**	**83** **183**	**86** **190**	**89** **196**	**92** **203**	**95** **209**	**98** **216**	**101** **223**	**104** **229**	**107** **236**	**110** **243**	**113** **249**	**116** **256**	**119** **262**
13.3	13.8	14.3	14.8	15.4	15.9	16.4	16.9	17.4	17.9	18.5	19.0	19.5	20.0	20.5
9.7	10.0	10.4	10.8	11.2	11.5	11.9	12.3	12.7	13.0	13.4	13.8	14.2	14.6	14.9
5.3	5.5	5.8	6.0	6.2	6.4	6.6	6.8	7.0	7.2	7.4	7.6	7.8	8.0	8.2
5.9	6.1	6.4	6.6	6.8	7.1	7.3	7.5	7.8	8.0	8.2	8.5	8.7	8.9	9.1
6.0	6.2	6.4	6.7	6.9	7.1	7.4	7.6	7.8	8.1	8.3	8.5	8.8	9.0	9.2
6.3	6.5	6.7	7.0	7.2	7.5	7.7	8.0	8.2	8.4	8.7	8.9	9.2	9.4	9.7
6.5	6.8	7.1	7.3	7.6	7.8	8.1	8.3	8.6	8.8	9.1	9.4	9.6	9.9	10.1
5.4	5.6	5.8	6.0	6.2	6.4	6.7	6.9	7.1	7.3	7.5	7.7	7.9	8.1	8.3
5.4	5.6	5.8	6.0	6.2	6.4	6.7	6.9	7.1	7.3	7.5	7.7	7.9	8.1	8.3
9.4	9.8	10.2	10.5	10.9	11.3	11.6	12.0	12.4	12.7	13.1	13.5	13.8	14.2	14.6
5.4	5.6	5.8	6.0	6.2	6.4	6.7	6.9	7.1	7.3	7.5	7.7	7.9	8.1	8.3
13.5	14.0	14.5	15.1	15.6	16.1	16.6	17.2	17.7	18.2	18.7	19.3	19.8	20.3	20.8
9.4	9.8	10.2	10.5	10.9	11.3	11.6	12.0	12.4	12.7	13.1	13.5	13.8	14.2	14.6
9.4	9.8	10.2	10.5	10.9	11.3	11.6	12.0	12.4	12.7	13.1	13.5	13.8	14.2	14.6
13.5	14.0	14.5	15.1	15.6	16.1	16.6	17.2	17.7	18.2	18.7	19.3	19.8	20.3	20.8
2.7	2.8	2.9	3.0	3.1	3.2	3.3	3.4	3.6	3.7	3.8	3.9	4.0	4.1	4.2
3.3	3.5	3.6	3.7	3.8	4.0	4.1	4.2	4.4	4.5	4.6	4.8	4.9	5.0	5.1
3.9	4.1	4.2	4.4	4.5	4.7	4.9	5.0	5.2	5.3	5.5	5.6	5.8	5.9	6.1
4.6	4.8	5.0	5.1	5.3	5.5	5.7	5.8	6.0	6.2	6.4	6.6	6.7	6.9	7.1
7.6	7.9	8.2	8.5	8.8	9.1	9.4	9.7	10.0	10.2	10.5	10.8	11.1	11.4	11.7
10.9	11.3	11.7	12.1	12.6	13.0	13.4	13.8	14.2	14.7	15.1	15.5	15.9	16.4	16.8
11.8	12.3	12.7	13.2	13.7	14.1	14.6	15.0	15.5	16.0	16.4	16.9	17.3	17.8	18.3
2.7	2.8	2.9	3.0	3.1	3.2	3.3	3.4	3.5	3.6	3.7	3.9	4.0	4.1	4.2
3.4	3.5	3.6	3.8	3.9	4.0	4.2	4.3	4.4	4.6	4.7	4.8	4.9	5.1	5.2

Calories Expended by Body Weight

| | | | | | Your Body Weight | | | | |
Activity	kg 50 lb 110	53 117	56 123	59 130	62 137	65 143	68 150	71 157	74 163
Standing (cont.)									
Light work (bartending, clerking, pumping gas, changing lightbulb)	2.2	2.3	2.5	2.6	2.7	2.8	3.0	3.1	3.2
Light/moderate work (assembling/ repairing heavy parts, welding, stocking shelves, patient care)	2.6	2.8	2.9	3.1	3.3	3.4	3.6	3.7	3.9
Moderate (assembling at fast rate)	3.1	3.2	3.4	3.6	3.8	4.0	4.2	4.3	4.5
Moderate/heavy (lifting more than 50 lb)	3.5	3.7	3.9	4.1	4.3	4.6	4.8	5.0	5.2
Packing/unpacking boxes, occasional lifting of household items, light to moderate effort	3.1	3.2	3.4	3.6	3.8	4.0	4.2	4.3	4.5
Playing with child—light	2.5	2.6	2.7	2.9	3.0	3.2	3.3	3.5	3.6
Reading	1.6	1.7	1.8	1.9	2.0	2.0	2.1	2.2	2.3
Shopping (nongrocery)	1.8	1.9	2.0	2.1	2.2	2.3	2.4	2.5	2.6
Standing quietly (in a line)	1.1	1.1	1.2	1.2	1.3	1.4	1.4	1.5	1.6
Talking	1.6	1.7	1.8	1.9	2.0	2.0	2.1	2.2	2.3
Steel Mill									
Fettling	4.4	4.6	4.9	5.2	5.4	5.7	6.0	6.2	6.5
Forging	4.8	5.1	5.4	5.7	6.0	6.3	6.5	6.8	7.1
Hand rolling	7.0	7.4	7.8	8.3	8.7	9.1	9.5	9.9	10.4
Merchant mill rolling	7.0	7.4	7.8	8.3	8.7	9.1	9.5	9.9	10.4
Removing slag	9.6	10.2	10.8	11.4	11.9	12.5	13.1	13.7	14.2
Tending furnace	6.6	7.0	7.4	7.7	8.1	8.5	8.9	9.3	9.7
Tipping molds	4.8	5.1	5.4	5.7	6.0	6.3	6.5	6.8	7.1
Working in general	7.0	7.4	7.8	8.3	8.7	9.1	9.5	9.9	10.4
Stretching (General)	3.5	3.7	3.9	4.1	4.3	4.6	4.8	5.0	5.2
Surfing (Body or Board, Pleasure or Competition)	3.2	3.3	3.5	3.7	3.9	4.1	4.3	4.5	4.7
Sweeping (Garage, Sidewalk, Outside)	3.5	3.7	3.9	4.1	4.3	4.6	4.8	5.0	5.2
Swimming—Backstroke									
Competition	7.4	7.9	8.3	8.8	9.2	9.7	10.1	10.6	11.0
General	7.0	7.4	7.8	8.3	8.7	9.1	9.5	9.9	10.4

Calories Expended by Body Weight

Your Body Weight

77 170	80 176	83 183	86 190	89 196	92 203	95 209	98 216	101 223	104 229	107 236	110 243	113 249	116 256	119 262
3.4	3.5	3.6	3.8	3.9	4.0	4.2	4.3	4.4	4.6	4.7	4.8	4.9	5.1	5.2
4.0	4.2	4.4	4.5	4.7	4.8	5.0	5.1	5.3	5.5	5.6	5.8	5.9	6.1	6.2
4.7	4.9	5.1	5.3	5.5	5.6	5.8	6.0	6.2	6.4	6.6	6.7	6.9	7.1	7.3
5.4	5.6	5.8	6.0	6.2	6.4	6.7	6.9	7.1	7.3	7.5	7.7	7.9	8.1	8.3
4.7	4.9	5.1	5.3	5.5	5.6	5.8	6.0	6.2	6.4	6.6	6.7	6.9	7.1	7.3
3.8	3.9	4.1	4.2	4.4	4.5	4.7	4.8	4.9	5.1	5.2	5.4	5.5	5.7	5.8
2.4	2.5	2.6	2.7	2.8	2.9	3.0	3.1	3.2	3.3	3.4	3.5	3.6	3.7	3.7
2.7	2.8	2.9	3.0	3.1	3.2	3.3	3.4	3.5	3.6	3.7	3.9	4.0	4.1	4.2
1.6	1.7	1.7	1.8	1.9	1.9	2.0	2.1	2.1	2.2	2.2	2.3	2.4	2.4	2.5
2.4	2.5	2.6	2.7	2.8	2.9	3.0	3.1	3.2	3.3	3.4	3.5	3.6	3.7	3.7
6.7	7.0	7.3	7.5	7.8	8.1	8.3	8.6	8.8	9.1	9.4	9.6	9.9	10.2	10.4
7.4	7.7	8.0	8.3	8.6	8.9	9.1	9.4	9.7	10.0	10.3	10.6	10.9	11.2	11.5
10.8	11.2	11.6	12.0	12.5	12.9	13.3	13.7	14.1	14.6	15.0	15.4	15.8	16.2	16.7
10.8	11.2	11.6	12.0	12.5	12.9	13.3	13.7	14.1	14.6	15.0	15.4	15.8	16.2	16.7
14.8	15.4	16.0	16.6	17.1	17.7	18.3	18.9	19.4	20.0	20.6	21.2	21.8	22.3	22.9
10.1	10.5	10.9	11.3	11.7	12.1	12.5	12.9	13.3	13.7	14.0	14.4	14.8	15.2	15.6
7.4	7.7	8.0	8.3	8.6	8.9	9.1	9.4	9.7	10.0	10.3	10.6	10.9	11.2	11.5
10.8	11.2	11.6	12.0	12.5	12.9	13.3	13.7	14.1	14.6	15.0	15.4	15.8	16.2	16.7
5.4	5.6	5.8	6.0	6.2	6.4	6.7	6.9	7.1	7.3	7.5	7.7	7.9	8.1	8.3
4.9	5.0	5.2	5.4	5.6	5.8	6.0	6.2	6.4	6.6	6.7	6.9	7.1	7.3	7.5
5.4	5.6	5.8	6.0	6.2	6.4	6.7	6.9	7.1	7.3	7.5	7.7	7.9	8.1	8.3
11.5	11.9	12.3	12.8	13.2	13.7	14.1	14.6	15.0	15.5	15.9	16.4	16.8	17.3	17.7
10.8	11.2	11.6	12.0	12.5	12.9	13.3	13.7	14.1	14.6	15.0	15.4	15.8	16.2	16.7

Calories Expended by Body Weight

Activity	kg 50 lb 110	53 117	56 123	59 130	62 137	65 143	68 150	71 157	74 163
Swimming—Breaststroke									
Competition	9.2	9.7	10.3	10.8	11.4	11.9	12.5	13.0	13.6
General	8.8	9.3	9.8	10.3	10.9	11.4	11.9	12.4	13.0
Swimming—Butterfly									
Competition	10.1	10.7	11.3	11.9	12.5	13.1	13.7	14.3	14.9
General	9.6	10.2	10.8	11.4	11.9	12.5	13.1	13.7	14.2
Swimming—Crawl									
Fast (75 yards/min.), vigorous effort	9.6	10.2	10.8	11.4	11.9	12.5	13.1	13.7	14.2
Slow (50 yards/min.), light/moderate effort	7.0	7.4	7.8	8.3	8.7	9.1	9.5	9.9	10.4
Swimming—Freestyle Laps									
Fast, maximal effort, competition, disabled athletes (walking with technical aid, polio, cerebral palsy), women	11.6	12.3	13.0	13.7	14.4	15.1	15.8	16.5	17.2
Fast, maximal effort, competition, disabled athletes (walking with technical aid, polio, cerebral palsy), men	10.7	11.3	11.9	12.6	13.2	13.9	14.5	15.1	15.8
Fast, maximal effort, competition, wheelchair-bound athletes, women	9.5	10.1	10.6	11.2	11.8	12.4	12.9	13.5	14.1
Fast, maximal effort, competition, wheelchair-bound athletes, men	10.1	10.7	11.3	11.9	12.5	13.1	13.7	14.3	14.9
Fast, vigorous effort, competition	9.2	9.7	10.3	10.8	11.4	11.9	12.5	13.0	13.6
Fast, vigorous effort, recreation	8.8	9.3	9.8	10.3	10.9	11.4	11.9	12.4	13.0
Slow, light or moderate effort	7.0	7.4	7.8	8.3	8.7	9.1	9.5	9.9	10.4
Swimming—General									
Lake, river, home pool (leisure)	5.3	5.6	5.9	6.2	6.5	6.8	7.1	7.5	7.8
Mini Gym Swim Bench, 41 strokes/min. (very slow)	13.1	13.9	14.7	15.4	16.2	17.0	17.8	18.6	19.4
Mini Gym Swim Bench, 43 strokes/min. (slow)	15.0	15.9	16.8	17.7	18.6	19.5	20.3	21.2	22.1

Calories Expended by Body Weight

Your Body Weight

77	80	83	86	89	92	95	98	101	104	107	110	113	116	119
170	176	183	190	196	203	209	216	223	229	236	243	249	256	262

| 14.1 | 14.7 | 15.3 | 15.8 | 16.4 | 16.9 | 17.5 | 18.0 | 18.6 | 19.1 | 19.7 | 20.2 | 20.8 | 21.3 | 21.9 |
| 13.5 | 14.0 | 14.5 | 15.1 | 15.6 | 16.1 | 16.6 | 17.2 | 17.7 | 18.2 | 18.7 | 19.3 | 19.8 | 20.3 | 20.8 |

| 15.5 | 16.1 | 16.7 | 17.3 | 17.9 | 18.5 | 19.1 | 19.7 | 20.3 | 20.9 | 21.5 | 22.1 | 22.7 | 23.3 | 23.9 |
| 14.8 | 15.4 | 16.0 | 16.6 | 17.1 | 17.7 | 18.3 | 18.9 | 19.4 | 20.0 | 20.6 | 21.2 | 21.8 | 22.3 | 22.9 |

| 14.8 | 15.4 | 16.0 | 16.6 | 17.1 | 17.7 | 18.3 | 18.9 | 19.4 | 20.0 | 20.6 | 21.2 | 21.8 | 22.3 | 22.9 |

| 10.8 | 11.2 | 11.6 | 12.0 | 12.5 | 12.9 | 13.3 | 13.7 | 14.1 | 14.6 | 15.0 | 15.4 | 15.8 | 16.2 | 16.7 |

| 17.9 | 18.6 | 19.3 | 20.0 | 20.7 | 21.3 | 22.0 | 22.7 | 23.4 | 24.1 | 24.8 | 25.5 | 26.2 | 26.9 | 27.6 |

| 16.4 | 17.1 | 17.7 | 18.3 | 19.0 | 19.6 | 20.2 | 20.9 | 21.5 | 22.2 | 22.8 | 23.4 | 24.1 | 24.7 | 25.4 |

| 14.6 | 15.2 | 15.8 | 16.3 | 16.9 | 17.5 | 18.1 | 18.6 | 19.2 | 19.8 | 20.3 | 20.9 | 21.5 | 22.0 | 22.6 |

| 15.5 | 16.1 | 16.7 | 17.3 | 17.9 | 18.5 | 19.2 | 19.8 | 20.4 | 21.0 | 21.6 | 22.2 | 22.8 | 23.4 | 24.0 |

14.1	14.7	15.3	15.8	16.4	16.9	17.5	18.0	18.6	19.1	19.7	20.2	20.8	21.3	21.9
13.5	14.0	14.5	15.1	15.6	16.1	16.6	17.2	17.7	18.2	18.7	19.3	19.8	20.3	20.8
10.8	11.2	11.6	12.0	12.5	12.9	13.3	13.7	14.1	14.6	15.0	15.4	15.8	16.2	16.7

| 8.1 | 8.4 | 8.7 | 9.0 | 9.3 | 9.7 | 10.0 | 10.3 | 10.6 | 10.9 | 11.2 | 11.6 | 11.9 | 12.2 | 12.5 |
| 20.2 | 20.9 | 21.7 | 22.5 | 23.3 | 24.1 | 24.9 | 25.7 | 26.4 | 27.2 | 28.0 | 28.8 | 29.6 | 30.4 | 31.2 |

| 23.0 | 23.9 | 24.8 | 25.7 | 26.6 | 27.5 | 28.4 | 29.3 | 30.2 | 31.1 | 32.0 | 32.9 | 33.8 | 34.7 | 35.6 |

Calories Expended by Body Weight

Activity	kg 50 lb 110	53 117	56 123	59 130	62 137	65 143	68 150	71 157	74 163
Swimming—General (cont.)									
Mini Gym Swim Bench, 45 strokes/min. (freely chosen)	16.9	17.9	18.9	19.9	20.9	22.0	23.0	24.0	25.0
Mini Gym Swim Bench, 48 strokes/min. (fast)	16.3	17.3	18.2	19.2	20.2	21.2	22.1	23.1	24.1
Mini Gym Swim Bench, 51 strokes/min. (very fast)	15.3	16.2	17.1	18.0	18.9	19.8	20.7	21.7	22.6
Ocean, competition (Ironman, triathlon)	10.1	10.7	11.3	11.9	12.5	13.1	13.7	14.3	14.9
Ocean, recreational	6.0	6.3	6.7	7.0	7.4	7.7	8.1	8.4	8.8
Swimming—Sidestroke	7.0	7.4	7.8	8.3	8.7	9.1	9.5	9.9	10.4
Swimming—Synchronized	7.0	7.4	7.8	8.3	8.7	9.1	9.5	9.9	10.4
Swimming—Treading Water									
Fast, vigorous effort	8.8	9.3	9.8	10.3	10.9	11.4	11.9	12.4	13.0
Moderate effort	3.5	3.7	3.9	4.1	4.3	4.6	4.8	5.0	5.2
Table Tennis (Ping-Pong)	3.5	3.7	3.9	4.1	4.3	4.6	4.8	5.0	5.2
Tae Kwon Do	8.2	8.7	9.2	9.7	10.2	10.7	11.2	11.7	12.2
Tai Chi									
Skilled performers	3.6	3.8	4.0	4.2	4.4	4.7	4.9	5.1	5.3
Unskilled performers	2.2	2.3	2.4	2.6	2.7	2.8	3.0	3.1	3.2
Tailoring									
Cutting	2.2	2.3	2.5	2.6	2.7	2.8	3.0	3.1	3.2
General	2.2	2.3	2.5	2.6	2.7	2.8	3.0	3.1	3.2
Hand sewing	1.8	1.9	2.0	2.1	2.2	2.3	2.4	2.5	2.6
Machine sewing	2.2	2.3	2.5	2.6	2.7	2.8	3.0	3.1	3.2
Pressing	3.5	3.7	3.9	4.1	4.3	4.6	4.8	5.0	5.2
Tennis									
Doubles, recreational	6.1	6.5	6.9	7.2	7.6	8.0	8.3	8.7	9.1
General	6.1	6.5	6.9	7.2	7.6	8.0	8.3	8.7	9.1
Singles, competition	8.1	8.5	9.0	9.5	10.0	10.5	10.9	11.4	11.9
Singles, recreational	7.0	7.4	7.8	8.3	8.7	9.1	9.5	9.9	10.4

Calories Expended by Body Weight

Your Body Weight

77 170	80 176	83 183	86 190	89 196	92 203	95 209	98 216	101 223	104 229	107 236	110 243	113 249	116 256	119 262
26.0	27.0	28.0	29.0	30.1	31.1	32.1	33.1	34.1	35.1	36.1	37.2	38.2	39.2	40.2
25.1	26.0	27.0	28.0	29.0	29.9	30.9	31.9	32.9	33.9	34.8	35.8	36.8	37.8	38.7
23.5	24.4	25.3	26.2	27.1	28.1	29.0	29.9	30.8	31.7	32.6	33.6	34.5	35.4	36.3
15.5	16.1	16.7	17.3	17.9	18.5	19.1	19.7	20.3	20.9	21.5	22.1	22.7	23.3	23.9
9.2	9.5	9.9	10.2	10.6	10.9	11.3	11.7	12.0	12.4	12.7	13.1	13.4	13.8	14.2
10.8	11.2	11.6	12.0	12.5	12.9	13.3	13.7	14.1	14.6	15.0	15.4	15.8	16.2	16.7
10.8	11.2	11.6	12.0	12.5	12.9	13.3	13.7	14.1	14.6	15.0	15.4	15.8	16.2	16.7
13.5	14.0	14.5	15.1	15.6	16.1	16.6	17.2	17.7	18.2	18.7	19.3	19.8	20.3	20.8
5.4	5.6	5.8	6.0	6.2	6.4	6.7	6.9	7.1	7.3	7.5	7.7	7.9	8.1	8.3
5.4	5.6	5.8	6.0	6.2	6.4	6.7	6.9	7.1	7.3	7.5	7.7	7.9	8.1	8.3
12.7	13.2	13.7	14.1	14.6	15.1	15.6	16.1	16.6	17.1	17.6	18.1	18.6	19.1	19.6
5.5	5.7	5.9	6.2	6.4	6.6	6.8	7.0	7.2	7.4	7.7	7.9	8.1	8.3	8.5
3.4	3.5	3.6	3.7	3.9	4.0	4.1	4.3	4.4	4.5	4.7	4.8	4.9	5.1	5.2
3.4	3.5	3.6	3.8	3.9	4.0	4.2	4.3	4.4	4.6	4.7	4.8	4.9	5.1	5.2
3.4	3.5	3.6	3.8	3.9	4.0	4.2	4.3	4.4	4.6	4.7	4.8	4.9	5.1	5.2
2.7	2.8	2.9	3.0	3.1	3.2	3.3	3.4	3.5	3.6	3.7	3.9	4.0	4.1	4.2
3.4	3.5	3.6	3.8	3.9	4.0	4.2	4.3	4.4	4.6	4.7	4.8	4.9	5.1	5.2
5.4	5.6	5.8	6.0	6.2	6.4	6.7	6.9	7.1	7.3	7.5	7.7	7.9	8.1	8.3
9.4	9.8	10.2	10.5	10.9	11.3	11.6	12.0	12.4	12.7	13.1	13.5	13.8	14.2	14.6
9.4	9.8	10.2	10.5	10.9	11.3	11.6	12.0	12.4	12.7	13.1	13.5	13.8	14.2	14.6
12.4	12.9	13.4	13.8	14.3	14.8	15.3	15.8	16.3	16.7	17.2	17.7	18.2	18.7	19.2
10.8	11.2	11.6	12.0	12.5	12.9	13.3	13.7	14.1	14.6	15.0	15.4	15.8	16.2	16.7

Calories Expended by Body Weight

Activity	kg lb	50 110	53 117	56 123	59 130	62 137	65 143	68 150	71 157	74 163
Theater (Actor, Craft Shop, Stagehand)		2.6	2.8	2.9	3.1	3.3	3.4	3.6	3.7	3.9
Trampolining (Recreational)		3.1	3.2	3.4	3.6	3.8	4.0	4.2	4.3	4.5
Triathalon—Competition										
Cycling, 55-miles (36% of max aerobic capacity)		5.1	5.4	5.7	6.0	6.3	6.7	7.0	7.3	7.6
Running, 12.4 miles (38% of max aerobic capacity)		5.9	6.3	6.6	7.0	7.3	7.7	8.1	8.4	8.8
Swimming, 1 mile (68% of max aerobic capacity)		7.8	8.2	8.7	9.2	9.6	10.1	10.6	11.0	11.5
Trombone Playing		3.1	3.2	3.4	3.6	3.8	4.0	4.2	4.3	4.5
Trumpet Playing		2.2	2.3	2.5	2.6	2.7	2.8	3.0	3.1	3.2
TV Reporting ("On-Air," Sitting)		1.5	1.6	1.7	1.8	1.8	1.9	2.0	2.1	2.2
Typing (Electric, Manual, or Computer)		1.3	1.4	1.5	1.5	1.6	1.7	1.8	1.9	1.9
Unicycling (Hard Surface)		4.4	4.6	4.9	5.2	5.4	5.7	6.0	6.2	6.5
Violin Playing		2.2	2.3	2.5	2.6	2.7	2.8	3.0	3.1	3.2
Volleyball										
Beach, competition		7.7	8.2	8.6	9.1	9.5	10.0	10.5	10.9	11.4
Beach, recreational		6.1	6.5	6.9	7.2	7.6	8.0	8.3	8.7	9.1
General, recreational (6- to 9-member team)		2.6	2.8	2.9	3.1	3.3	3.4	3.6	3.7	3.9
Gymnasium, competition		3.5	3.7	3.9	4.1	4.3	4.6	4.8	5.0	5.2
No sand, competition (indoors, outdoors)		6.6	7.0	7.4	7.7	8.1	8.5	8.9	9.3	9.7
Wallyball, general		6.1	6.5	6.9	7.2	7.6	8.0	8.3	8.7	9.1
Water		2.6	2.8	2.9	3.1	3.3	3.4	3.6	3.7	3.9
Walking—General										
Less than 2 mph, on job (office), slow pace		1.8	1.9	2.0	2.1	2.2	2.3	2.4	2.5	2.6

Calories Expended by Body Weight

Your Body Weight

77 170	80 176	83 183	86 190	89 196	92 203	95 209	98 216	101 223	104 229	107 236	110 243	113 249	116 256	119 262
4.0	4.2	4.4	4.5	4.7	4.8	5.0	5.1	5.3	5.5	5.6	5.8	5.9	6.1	6.2
4.7	4.9	5.1	5.3	5.5	5.6	5.8	6.0	6.2	6.4	6.6	6.7	6.9	7.1	7.3
7.9	8.2	8.5	8.8	9.1	9.4	9.7	10.0	10.3	10.6	11.0	11.3	11.6	11.9	12.2
9.1	9.5	9.8	10.2	10.5	10.9	11.3	11.6	12.0	12.3	12.7	13.0	13.4	13.7	14.1
12.0	12.4	12.9	13.4	13.8	14.3	14.8	15.2	15.7	16.2	16.6	17.1	17.6	18.0	18.5
4.7	4.9	5.1	5.3	5.5	5.6	5.8	6.0	6.2	6.4	6.6	6.7	6.9	7.1	7.3
3.4	3.5	3.6	3.8	3.9	4.0	4.2	4.3	4.4	4.6	4.7	4.8	4.9	5.1	5.2
2.3	2.4	2.5	2.6	2.6	2.7	2.8	2.9	3.0	3.1	3.2	3.3	3.4	3.5	3.5
2.0	2.1	2.2	2.3	2.3	2.4	2.5	2.6	2.7	2.7	2.8	2.9	3.0	3.0	3.1
6.7	7.0	7.3	7.5	7.8	8.1	8.3	8.6	8.8	9.1	9.4	9.6	9.9	10.2	10.4
3.4	3.5	3.6	3.8	3.9	4.0	4.2	4.3	4.4	4.6	4.7	4.8	4.9	5.1	5.2
11.9	12.3	12.8	13.2	13.7	14.2	14.6	15.1	15.6	16.0	16.5	16.9	17.4	17.9	18.3
9.4	9.8	10.2	10.5	10.9	11.3	11.6	12.0	12.4	12.7	13.1	13.5	13.8	14.2	14.6
4.0	4.2	4.4	4.5	4.7	4.8	5.0	5.1	5.3	5.5	5.6	5.8	5.9	6.1	6.2
5.4	5.6	5.8	6.0	6.2	6.4	6.7	6.9	7.1	7.3	7.5	7.7	7.9	8.1	8.3
10.1	10.5	10.9	11.3	11.7	12.1	12.5	12.9	13.3	13.7	14.0	14.4	14.8	15.2	15.6
9.4	9.8	10.2	10.5	10.9	11.3	11.6	12.0	12.4	12.7	13.1	13.5	13.8	14.2	14.6
4.0	4.2	4.4	4.5	4.7	4.8	5.0	5.1	5.3	5.5	5.6	5.8	5.9	6.1	6.2
2.7	2.8	2.9	3.0	3.1	3.2	3.3	3.4	3.5	3.6	3.7	3.9	4.0	4.1	4.2

Calories Expended by Body Weight

Activity	kg 50 lb 110	53 117	56 123	59 130	62 137	65 143	68 150	71 157	74 163
Walking—General (cont.)									
2 mph, level, slow pace, firm surface	2.2	2.3	2.5	2.6	2.7	2.8	3.0	3.1	3.2
2.5 mph, downhill	2.6	2.8	2.9	3.1	3.3	3.4	3.6	3.7	3.9
2.5 mph, firm surface	2.6	2.8	2.9	3.1	3.3	3.4	3.6	3.7	3.9
2.5 mph, slow pace, carrying light objects less than 25 lb	2.6	2.8	2.9	3.1	3.3	3.4	3.6	3.7	3.9
3 mph, level, moderate pace, firm surface	3.1	3.2	3.4	3.6	3.8	4.0	4.2	4.3	4.5
3 mph, moderate pace, carrying light objects less than 25 lb	3.5	3.7	3.9	4.1	4.3	4.6	4.8	5.0	5.2
3 mph, on job (office), moderate pace	3.1	3.2	3.4	3.6	3.8	4.0	4.2	4.3	4.5
3.5 mph, brisk pace and carrying objects less than 25 lb	3.9	4.2	4.4	4.6	4.9	5.1	5.4	5.6	5.8
3.5 mph, carrying 1 lb weights	3.9	4.1	4.3	4.5	4.8	5.0	5.2	5.5	5.7
3.5 mph, carrying 5 lb weights	4.6	4.9	5.2	5.4	5.7	6.0	6.3	6.5	6.8
3.5 mph, level, brisk pace, firm surface	3.5	3.7	3.9	4.1	4.3	4.6	4.8	5.0	5.2
3.5 mph, on job (office), brisk pace	3.5	3.7	3.9	4.1	4.3	4.6	4.8	5.0	5.2
3.5 mph, uphill	5.3	5.6	5.9	6.2	6.5	6.8	7.1	7.5	7.8
4 mph, level, brisk pace, firm surface	3.5	3.7	3.9	4.1	4.3	4.6	4.8	5.0	5.2
4.5 mph, level, very brisk pace, firm surface	3.9	4.2	4.4	4.6	4.9	5.1	5.4	5.6	5.8
Backward, 4 mph (15 min./mile)	8.3	8.8	9.3	9.8	10.3	10.8	11.3	11.8	12.3
Carrying objects 25 to 49 lb	4.4	4.6	4.9	5.2	5.4	5.7	6.0	6.2	6.5
Carrying objects 50 to 74 lb	5.7	6.0	6.4	6.7	7.1	7.4	7.7	8.1	8.4
Carrying objects 75 to 99 lb	6.6	7.0	7.4	7.7	8.1	8.5	8.9	9.3	9.7
Carrying objects more than 99 lb	7.4	7.9	8.3	8.8	9.2	9.7	10.1	10.6	11.0
Carrying Heavy Hands (2 lb each), 3 mph, 110 pumps/min., each pump 24–42 in. above shoulder height	5.9	6.3	6.6	7.0	7.4	7.7	8.1	8.4	8.8
Carrying Heavy Hands (2 lb each), 4 mph, 130 pumps/min., each pump well above shoulder height	8.8	9.3	9.8	10.3	10.9	11.4	11.9	12.4	13.0

Calories Expended by Body Weight

Your Body Weight

77 170	80 176	83 183	86 190	89 196	92 203	95 209	98 216	101 223	104 229	107 236	110 243	113 249	116 256	119 262
3.4	3.5	3.6	3.8	3.9	4.0	4.2	4.3	4.4	4.6	4.7	4.8	4.9	5.1	5.2
4.0	4.2	4.4	4.5	4.7	4.8	5.0	5.1	5.3	5.5	5.6	5.8	5.9	6.1	6.2
4.0	4.2	4.4	4.5	4.7	4.8	5.0	5.1	5.3	5.5	5.6	5.8	5.9	6.1	6.2
4.0	4.2	4.4	4.5	4.7	4.8	5.0	5.1	5.3	5.5	5.6	5.8	5.9	6.1	6.2
4.7	4.9	5.1	5.3	5.5	5.6	5.8	6.0	6.2	6.4	6.6	6.7	6.9	7.1	7.3
5.4	5.6	5.8	6.0	6.2	6.4	6.7	6.9	7.1	7.3	7.5	7.7	7.9	8.1	8.3
4.7	4.9	5.1	5.3	5.5	5.6	5.8	6.0	6.2	6.4	6.6	6.7	6.9	7.1	7.3
6.1	6.3	6.5	6.8	7.0	7.2	7.5	7.7	8.0	8.2	8.4	8.7	8.9	9.1	9.4
5.9	6.2	6.4	6.6	6.9	7.1	7.3	7.5	7.8	8.0	8.2	8.5	8.7	8.9	9.2
7.1	7.4	7.6	7.9	8.2	8.5	8.7	9.0	9.3	9.6	9.8	10.1	10.4	10.7	11.0
5.4	5.6	5.8	6.0	6.2	6.4	6.7	6.9	7.1	7.3	7.5	7.7	7.9	8.1	8.3
5.4	5.6	5.8	6.0	6.2	6.4	6.7	6.9	7.1	7.3	7.5	7.7	7.9	8.1	8.3
8.1	8.4	8.7	9.0	9.3	9.7	10.0	10.3	10.6	10.9	11.2	11.6	11.9	12.2	12.5
5.4	5.6	5.8	6.0	6.2	6.4	6.7	6.9	7.1	7.3	7.5	7.7	7.9	8.1	8.3
6.1	6.3	6.5	6.8	7.0	7.2	7.5	7.7	8.0	8.2	8.4	8.7	8.9	9.1	9.4
12.8	13.3	13.8	14.3	14.8	15.3	15.8	16.3	16.8	17.3	17.8	18.3	18.8	19.3	19.8
6.7	7.0	7.3	7.5	7.8	8.1	8.3	8.6	8.8	9.1	9.4	9.6	9.9	10.2	10.4
8.8	9.1	9.4	9.8	10.1	10.5	10.8	11.1	11.5	11.8	12.2	12.5	12.9	13.2	13.5
10.1	10.5	10.9	11.3	11.7	12.1	12.5	12.9	13.3	13.7	14.0	14.4	14.8	15.2	15.6
11.5	11.9	12.3	12.8	13.2	13.7	14.1	14.6	15.0	15.5	15.9	16.4	16.8	17.3	17.7
9.1	9.5	9.8	10.2	10.6	10.9	11.3	11.6	12.0	12.3	12.7	13.1	13.4	13.8	14.1
13.5	14.0	14.5	15.1	15.6	16.1	16.6	17.2	17.7	18.2	18.7	19.3	19.8	20.3	20.8

Calories Expended by Body Weight

Activity	kg	50	53	56	59	62	65	68	71	74
	lb	110	117	123	130	137	143	150	157	163

Walking—General (cont.)

Activity	50/110	53/117	56/123	59/130	62/137	65/143	68/150	71/157	74/163
Carrying Heavy Hands (3 lb each), 3.5 mph, 120 pumps/min., each pump 24 in. above shoulder height	8.6	9.1	9.6	10.1	10.6	11.1	11.7	12.2	12.7
Carrying Heavy Hands (3 lb each), 3.5 mph, 120 pumps/min., each pump 42 inches above shoulder height	8.6	9.1	9.7	10.2	10.7	11.2	11.7	12.2	12.8
Down stairs	2.6	2.8	2.9	3.1	3.3	3.4	3.6	3.7	3.9
Grass track	4.4	4.6	4.9	5.2	5.4	5.7	6.0	6.2	6.5
Less than 2.0 mph, level, strolling, household walking, very slow pace	1.8	1.9	2.0	2.1	2.2	2.3	2.4	2.5	2.6
Light, noncleaning (leaving house/shutting/locking doors, closing windows)	2.6	2.8	2.9	3.1	3.3	3.4	3.6	3.7	3.9
Normal pace, to work or class	3.5	3.7	3.9	4.1	4.3	4.6	4.8	5.0	5.2
Pleasure, work break, walking the dog	3.1	3.2	3.4	3.6	3.8	4.0	4.2	4.3	4.5
Shopping (nongrocery)	2.0	2.1	2.3	2.4	2.5	2.6	2.7	2.9	3.0
Up stairs, climbing ladder	7.0	7.4	7.8	8.3	8.7	9.1	9.5	9.9	10.4
Wearing 1 lb wrist weights, 60% of max heart rate	6.8	7.2	7.6	8.0	8.4	8.8	9.2	9.7	10.1
Wearing 1 lb wrist weights, 70% of max heart rate	7.8	8.2	8.7	9.2	9.6	10.1	10.6	11.0	11.5
Wearing 3 lb wrist weights, 60% of max heart rate	7.1	7.6	8.0	8.4	8.9	9.3	9.7	10.2	10.6
Wearing 3 lb wrist weights, 75% of max heart rate	8.1	8.6	9.1	9.6	10.1	10.6	11.1	11.5	12.0
Weighted with 10% body weight, 3.5 mph, women	3.9	4.1	4.3	4.6	4.8	5.0	5.3	5.5	5.7
Weighted with 10% body weight, 3.5 mph, men	4.0	4.3	4.5	4.7	5.0	5.2	5.5	5.7	6.0
Weighted with 10% body weight, 4 mph, women	4.7	5.0	5.2	5.5	5.8	6.1	6.4	6.6	6.9
Weighted with 10% body weight, 4 mph, men	5.3	5.6	6.0	6.3	6.6	6.9	7.2	7.6	7.9
Weighted with 20% body weight, 3.5 mph, women	4.3	4.6	4.9	5.1	5.4	5.7	5.9	6.2	6.4

Calories Expended by Body Weight

Your Body Weight

77 170	80 176	83 183	86 190	89 196	92 203	95 209	98 216	101 223	104 229	107 236	110 243	113 249	116 256	119 262
13.2	13.7	14.2	14.7	15.3	15.8	16.3	16.8	17.3	17.8	18.4	18.9	19.4	19.9	20.4
13.3	13.8	14.3	14.8	15.3	15.9	16.4	16.9	17.4	17.9	18.4	19.0	19.5	20.0	20.5
4.0	4.2	4.4	4.5	4.7	4.8	5.0	5.1	5.3	5.5	5.6	5.8	5.9	6.1	6.2
6.7	7.0	7.3	7.5	7.8	8.1	8.3	8.6	8.8	9.1	9.4	9.6	9.9	10.2	10.4
2.7	2.8	2.9	3.0	3.1	3.2	3.3	3.4	3.5	3.6	3.7	3.9	4.0	4.1	4.2
4.0	4.2	4.4	4.5	4.7	4.8	5.0	5.1	5.3	5.5	5.6	5.8	5.9	6.1	6.2
5.4	5.6	5.8	6.0	6.2	6.4	6.7	6.9	7.1	7.3	7.5	7.7	7.9	8.1	8.3
4.7	4.9	5.1	5.3	5.5	5.6	5.8	6.0	6.2	6.4	6.6	6.7	6.9	7.1	7.3
3.1	3.2	3.3	3.5	3.6	3.7	3.8	3.9	4.1	4.2	4.3	4.4	4.5	4.7	4.8
10.8	11.2	11.6	12.0	12.5	12.9	13.3	13.7	14.1	14.6	15.0	15.4	15.8	16.2	16.7
10.5	10.9	11.3	11.7	12.1	12.5	12.9	13.3	13.7	14.1	14.5	15.0	15.4	15.8	16.2
12.0	12.4	12.9	13.4	13.8	14.3	14.8	15.2	15.7	16.2	16.6	17.1	17.6	18.0	18.5
11.0	11.4	11.9	12.3	12.7	13.2	13.6	14.0	14.4	14.9	15.3	15.7	16.2	16.6	17.0
12.5	13.0	13.5	14.0	14.5	15.0	15.4	15.9	16.4	16.9	17.4	17.9	18.4	18.9	19.3
6.0	6.2	6.4	6.7	6.9	7.1	7.3	7.6	7.8	8.0	8.3	8.5	8.7	9.0	9.2
6.2	6.4	6.7	6.9	7.2	7.4	7.6	7.9	8.1	8.4	8.6	8.9	9.1	9.3	9.6
7.2	7.5	7.8	8.0	8.3	8.6	8.9	9.2	9.4	9.7	10.0	10.3	10.6	10.8	11.1
8.2	8.5	8.8	9.2	9.5	9.8	10.1	10.4	10.8	11.1	11.4	11.7	12.0	12.4	12.7
6.7	7.0	7.2	7.5	7.7	8.0	8.3	8.5	8.8	9.0	9.3	9.6	9.8	10.1	10.4

Calories Expended by Body Weight

					Your Body Weight				
Activity	**kg** **lb**	**50** **110**	**53** **117**	**56** **123**	**59** **130**	**62** **137**	**65** **143**	**68** **150**	**71** **157**	**74** **163**

Activity	50/110	53/117	56/123	59/130	62/137	65/143	68/150	71/157	74/163
Walking—General (cont.)									
Weighted with 20% body weight, 3.5 mph, men	4.5	4.8	5.0	5.3	5.6	5.8	6.1	6.4	6.7
Weighted with 20% body weight, 4 mph, women	5.2	5.5	5.8	6.1	6.4	6.7	7.0	7.3	7.7
Weighted with 20% body weight, 4 mph, men	5.8	6.2	6.5	6.9	7.2	7.6	7.9	8.3	8.6
Weighted with 30% body weight, 3.5 mph, women	4.5	4.8	5.0	5.3	5.6	5.8	6.1	6.4	6.7
Weighted with 30% body weight, 3.5 mph, men	4.9	5.2	5.5	5.8	6.0	6.3	6.6	6.9	7.2
Weighted with 30% body weight, 4 mph, women	5.3	5.6	5.9	6.2	6.5	6.8	7.1	7.5	7.8
Weighted with 30% body weight, 4 mph, men	6.3	6.7	7.1	7.4	7.8	8.2	8.6	8.9	9.3
Weighted with 40% body weight, 3.5 mph, women	4.9	5.2	5.5	5.8	6.1	6.4	6.7	7.0	7.3
Weighted with 40% body weight, 3.5 mph, men	5.1	5.4	5.7	6.1	6.4	6.7	7.0	7.3	7.6
Weighted with 40% body weight, 4 mph, women	6.2	6.6	6.9	7.3	7.7	8.1	8.4	8.8	9.2
Weighted with 40% body weight, 4 mph, men	6.7	7.2	7.6	8.0	8.4	8.8	9.2	9.6	10.0
Walking—with Crutches									
General	3.5	3.7	3.9	4.1	4.3	4.6	4.8	5.0	5.2
1.1 mph, level	2.7	2.9	3.0	3.2	3.4	3.5	3.7	3.8	4.0
1.5 mph, level	3.4	3.6	3.8	4.0	4.2	4.4	4.7	4.9	5.1
1.9 mph, level	3.6	3.9	4.1	4.3	4.5	4.7	5.0	5.2	5.4
2.3 mph, level	4.5	4.8	5.0	5.3	5.6	5.8	6.1	6.4	6.7
2.6 mph, level	4.9	5.2	5.5	5.8	6.1	6.4	6.7	7.0	7.3
3.0 mph, level	6.1	6.5	6.8	7.2	7.6	7.9	8.3	8.7	9.0
1.5 mph, 5% grade	3.9	4.1	4.4	4.6	4.8	5.1	5.3	5.5	5.8
2.2 mph, 5% grade	5.5	5.8	6.1	6.4	6.8	7.1	7.4	7.7	8.1
Walking—Race									
6.2 mph, competitive racewalkers	11.3	11.9	12.6	13.3	14.0	14.6	15.3	16.0	16.7
6.8 mph, competitive racewalkers	11.9	12.6	13.3	14.0	14.7	15.4	16.1	16.9	17.6
7.5 mph, competitive racewalkers	12.3	13.0	13.7	14.5	15.2	15.9	16.7	17.4	18.1

Calories Expended by Body Weight

\						Your Body Weight								
77 **170**	**80** **176**	**83** **183**	**86** **190**	**89** **196**	**92** **203**	**95** **209**	**98** **216**	**101** **223**	**104** **229**	**107** **236**	**110** **243**	**113** **249**	**116** **256**	**119** **262**
6.9	7.2	7.5	7.7	8.0	8.3	8.5	8.8	9.1	9.4	9.6	9.9	10.2	10.4	10.7
8.0	8.3	8.6	8.9	9.2	9.5	9.8	10.1	10.4	10.8	11.1	11.4	11.7	12.0	12.3
9.0	9.3	9.7	10.0	10.4	10.7	11.1	11.4	11.8	12.1	12.5	12.8	13.2	13.5	13.9
6.9	7.2	7.5	7.7	8.0	8.3	8.5	8.8	9.1	9.4	9.6	9.9	10.2	10.4	10.7
7.5	7.8	8.1	8.4	8.7	9.0	9.3	9.6	9.8	10.1	10.4	10.7	11.0	11.3	11.6
8.1	8.4	8.7	9.0	9.3	9.7	10.0	10.3	10.6	10.9	11.2	11.6	11.9	12.2	12.5
9.7	10.1	10.5	10.8	11.2	11.6	12.0	12.3	12.7	13.1	13.5	13.9	14.2	14.6	15.0
7.6	7.9	8.2	8.5	8.8	9.0	9.3	9.6	9.9	10.2	10.5	10.8	11.1	11.4	11.7
7.9	8.2	8.5	8.8	9.1	9.4	9.7	10.0	10.4	10.7	11.0	11.3	11.6	11.9	12.2
9.6	9.9	10.3	10.7	11.0	11.4	11.8	12.2	12.5	12.9	13.3	13.6	14.0	14.4	14.8
10.4	10.8	11.2	11.6	12.0	12.4	12.8	13.2	13.6	14.0	14.4	14.8	15.2	15.7	16.1
5.4	5.6	5.8	6.0	6.2	6.4	6.7	6.9	7.1	7.3	7.5	7.7	7.9	8.1	8.3
4.2	4.3	4.5	4.7	4.8	5.0	5.1	5.3	5.5	5.6	5.8	5.9	6.1	6.3	6.4
5.3	5.5	5.7	5.9	6.1	6.3	6.5	6.7	6.9	7.1	7.3	7.5	7.7	7.9	8.1
5.6	5.8	6.1	6.3	6.5	6.7	6.9	7.2	7.4	7.6	7.8	8.0	8.2	8.5	8.7
6.9	7.2	7.5	7.7	8.0	8.3	8.5	8.8	9.1	9.4	9.6	9.9	10.2	10.4	10.7
7.5	7.8	8.1	8.4	8.7	9.0	9.3	9.6	9.9	10.2	10.5	10.8	11.1	11.4	11.7
9.4	9.8	10.1	10.5	10.9	11.2	11.6	12.0	12.3	12.7	13.1	13.4	13.8	14.1	14.5
6.0	6.2	6.5	6.7	6.9	7.2	7.4	7.6	7.9	8.1	8.4	8.6	8.8	9.1	9.3
8.4	8.7	9.0	9.4	9.7	10.0	10.4	10.7	11.0	11.3	11.7	12.0	12.3	12.6	13.0
17.3	18.0	18.7	19.4	20.0	20.7	21.4	22.1	22.7	23.4	24.1	24.8	25.4	26.1	26.8
18.3	19.0	19.7	20.4	21.1	21.8	22.6	23.3	24.0	24.7	25.4	26.1	26.8	27.5	28.3
18.9	19.6	20.3	21.1	21.8	22.5	23.3	24.0	24.7	25.5	26.2	27.0	27.7	28.4	29.2

Calories Expended by Body Weight

		Your Body Weight							
Activity	kg 50 lb 110	53 117	56 123	59 130	62 137	65 143	68 150	71 157	74 163
Walking—Race (cont.)									
8.1 mph, competitive racewalkers	13.0	13.8	14.6	15.3	16.1	16.9	17.7	18.5	19.2
8.7 mph, competitive racewalkers	13.4	14.3	15.1	15.9	16.7	17.5	18.3	19.1	19.9
Competition, 6 mph	9.6	10.2	10.8	11.4	11.9	12.5	13.1	13.7	14.2
Competition, 7 mph	11.4	12.1	12.7	13.4	14.1	14.8	15.5	16.2	16.8
Competition, 8 mph, men	14.9	15.8	16.7	17.6	18.4	19.3	20.2	21.1	22.0
Competition, 8 mph, women	14.0	14.8	15.7	16.5	17.4	18.2	19.0	19.9	20.7
Competition, 8.5 mph, men	15.8	16.7	17.6	18.6	19.5	20.5	21.4	22.4	23.3
Recreational	5.7	6.0	6.4	6.7	7.1	7.4	7.7	8.1	8.4
Walking—Treadmill (men and women)									
2 mph, level	2.7	2.9	3.1	3.2	3.4	3.5	3.7	3.9	4.0
2.5 mph, level	3.4	3.6	3.8	4.0	4.2	4.4	4.6	4.8	5.0
3 mph, level	4.0	4.2	4.5	4.7	4.9	5.2	5.4	5.7	5.9
3.5 mph, level	4.5	4.8	5.1	5.3	5.6	5.9	6.1	6.4	6.7
4 mph, level	5.1	5.5	5.8	6.1	6.4	6.7	7.0	7.3	7.6
3.4 mph, -3% grade	2.0	2.1	2.2	2.4	2.5	2.6	2.7	2.8	3.0
3.9 mph, -3% grade	2.7	2.9	3.0	3.2	3.4	3.5	3.7	3.8	4.0
Washing									
Dishes, standing	2.0	2.1	2.3	2.4	2.5	2.6	2.7	2.9	3.0
Dishes: clearing dishes from table, walking	2.0	2.1	2.3	2.4	2.5	2.6	2.7	2.9	3.0
Fences, walls	3.9	4.2	4.4	4.6	4.9	5.1	5.4	5.6	5.8
Standing (laundry, folding or hanging clothes, putting clothes in washer or dryer, packing suitcase)	1.8	1.9	2.0	2.1	2.2	2.3	2.4	2.5	2.6
Walking (putting away clothes, gathering clothes to pack, putting away laundry)	2.0	2.1	2.3	2.4	2.5	2.6	2.7	2.9	3.0
Washing and waxing sailboat hull, car, powerboat, airplane	3.9	4.2	4.4	4.6	4.9	5.1	5.4	5.6	5.8
Water Polo									
Competition	8.8	9.4	9.9	10.4	11.0	11.5	12.0	12.5	13.1
Recreational, moderate	6.6	7.0	7.4	7.7	8.1	8.5	8.9	9.3	9.7
Recreational, vigorous	8.8	9.3	9.8	10.3	10.9	11.4	11.9	12.4	13.0

Calories Expended by Body Weight

Your Body Weight

77 170	80 176	83 183	86 190	89 196	92 203	95 209	98 216	101 223	104 229	107 236	110 243	113 249	116 256	119 262
20.0	20.8	21.6	22.4	23.1	23.9	24.7	25.5	26.3	27.0	27.8	28.6	29.4	30.2	30.9
20.7	21.5	22.3	23.1	23.9	24.7	25.6	26.4	27.2	28.0	28.8	29.6	30.4	31.2	32.0
14.8	15.4	16.0	16.6	17.1	17.7	18.3	18.9	19.4	20.0	20.6	21.2	21.8	22.3	22.9
17.5	18.2	18.9	19.6	20.2	20.9	21.6	22.3	23.0	23.7	24.3	25.0	25.7	26.4	27.1
22.9	23.8	24.7	25.6	26.5	27.4	28.3	29.2	30.0	30.9	31.8	32.7	33.6	34.5	35.4
21.6	22.4	23.2	24.1	24.9	25.8	26.6	27.4	28.3	29.1	30.0	30.8	31.6	32.5	33.3
24.3	25.2	26.1	27.1	28.0	29.0	29.9	30.9	31.8	32.8	33.7	34.7	35.6	36.5	37.5
8.8	9.1	9.4	9.8	10.1	10.5	10.8	11.1	11.5	11.8	12.2	12.5	12.9	13.2	13.5
4.2	4.4	4.5	4.7	4.9	5.0	5.2	5.4	5.5	5.7	5.8	6.0	6.2	6.3	6.5
5.2	5.4	5.6	5.8	6.0	6.2	6.4	6.6	6.8	7.0	7.2	7.4	7.6	7.8	8.0
6.1	6.4	6.6	6.9	7.1	7.3	7.6	7.8	8.1	8.3	8.5	8.8	9.0	9.3	9.5
7.0	7.2	7.5	7.8	8.0	8.3	8.6	8.8	9.1	9.4	9.7	9.9	10.2	10.5	10.7
7.9	8.2	8.5	8.8	9.2	9.5	9.8	10.1	10.4	10.7	11.0	11.3	11.6	11.9	12.2
3.1	3.2	3.3	3.4	3.6	3.7	3.8	3.9	4.0	4.2	4.3	4.4	4.5	4.6	4.8
4.2	4.3	4.5	4.7	4.8	5.0	5.1	5.3	5.5	5.6	5.8	5.9	6.1	6.3	6.4
3.1	3.2	3.3	3.5	3.6	3.7	3.8	3.9	4.1	4.2	4.3	4.4	4.5	4.7	4.8
3.1	3.2	3.3	3.5	3.6	3.7	3.8	3.9	4.1	4.2	4.3	4.4	4.5	4.7	4.8
6.1	6.3	6.5	6.8	7.0	7.2	7.5	7.7	8.0	8.2	8.4	8.7	8.9	9.1	9.4
2.7	2.8	2.9	3.0	3.1	3.2	3.3	3.4	3.5	3.6	3.7	3.9	4.0	4.1	4.2
3.1	3.2	3.3	3.5	3.6	3.7	3.8	3.9	4.1	4.2	4.3	4.4	4.5	4.7	4.8
6.1	6.3	6.5	6.8	7.0	7.2	7.5	7.7	8.0	8.2	8.4	8.7	8.9	9.1	9.4
13.6	14.1	14.7	15.2	15.7	16.3	16.8	17.3	17.9	18.4	18.9	19.4	20.0	20.5	21.0
10.1	10.5	10.9	11.3	11.7	12.1	12.5	12.9	13.3	13.7	14.0	14.4	14.8	15.2	15.6
13.5	14.0	14.5	15.1	15.6	16.1	16.6	17.2	17.7	18.2	18.7	19.3	19.8	20.3	20.8

Calories Expended by Body Weight

Activity	kg lb	50 110	53 117	56 123	59 130	62 137	65 143	68 150	71 157	74 163
Weight Lifting— Body Builder Training		5.2	5.5	5.8	6.1	6.4	6.8	7.1	7.4	7.7
Weight Lifting—Olympic Lifts										
40% of 1-RM, dead lift		4.5	4.7	5.0	5.3	5.6	5.8	6.1	6.4	6.6
50% of 1-RM, dead lift		5.1	5.4	5.8	6.1	6.4	6.7	7.0	7.3	7.6
60% of 1-RM, dead lift		5.9	6.2	6.6	6.9	7.3	7.7	8.0	8.4	8.7
70% of 1-RM, dead lift		6.4	6.8	7.1	7.5	7.9	8.3	8.7	9.0	9.4
70% of 1-RM, clean and jerk		5.4	5.7	6.0	6.3	6.7	7.0	7.3	7.6	8.0
70% of 1-RM, snatch		3.7	4.0	4.2	4.4	4.6	4.9	5.1	5.3	5.5
85% of 1-RM, clean and jerk		6.5	6.9	7.3	7.6	8.0	8.4	8.8	9.2	9.6
85% of 1-RM, snatch		4.5	4.8	5.0	5.3	5.6	5.8	6.1	6.4	6.7
Weight Lifting—Power Lifting		5.0	5.3	5.6	5.9	6.2	6.6	6.9	7.2	7.5
Wheelchair Ergometry										
Backward, 15 watts		3.7	3.9	4.1	4.3	4.6	4.8	5.0	5.2	5.4
Backward, 20 watts		6.9	7.3	7.8	8.2	8.6	9.0	9.4	9.8	10.3
Backward, 25 watts		4.9	5.2	5.5	5.8	6.1	6.4	6.7	7.0	7.3
Backward, 30 watts		5.1	5.5	5.8	6.1	6.4	6.7	7.0	7.3	7.6
Forward, 15 watts		4.4	4.7	4.9	5.2	5.5	5.7	6.0	6.3	6.5
Forward, 20 watts		5.1	5.4	5.8	6.1	6.4	6.7	7.0	7.3	7.6
Forward, 25 watts		5.9	6.2	6.6	6.9	7.3	7.6	8.0	8.3	8.7
Forward, 30 watts		6.6	7.0	7.4	7.8	8.2	8.6	9.0	9.4	9.8
Whirlpool (Sitting and Relaxing)		0.9	1.0	1.0	1.1	1.1	1.2	1.2	1.3	1.3
Whitewater Rafting (Recreational)		4.4	4.6	4.9	5.2	5.4	5.7	6.0	6.2	6.5
Wind Surfing		3.5	3.7	3.9	4.1	4.3	4.6	4.8	5.0	5.2
Woodwind Playing		1.8	1.9	2.0	2.1	2.2	2.3	2.4	2.5	2.6
Wrestling (5 min./match)		7.3	7.7	8.1	8.6	9.0	9.4	9.9	10.3	10.7
Yoga		3.0	3.2	3.3	3.5	3.7	3.9	4.0	4.2	4.4

Calories Expended by Body Weight

Your Body Weight

77 170	80 176	83 183	86 190	89 196	92 203	95 209	98 216	101 223	104 229	107 236	110 243	113 249	116 256	119 262
8.0	8.3	8.6	8.9	9.3	9.6	9.9	10.2	10.5	10.8	11.1	11.4	11.7	12.1	12.4
6.9	7.2	7.4	7.7	8.0	8.2	8.5	8.8	9.0	9.3	9.6	9.9	10.1	10.4	10.7
7.9	8.2	8.5	8.8	9.1	9.5	9.8	10.1	10.4	10.7	11.0	11.3	11.6	11.9	12.2
9.1	9.4	9.8	10.1	10.5	10.8	11.2	11.5	11.9	12.2	12.6	13.0	13.3	13.7	14.0
9.8	10.2	10.6	11.0	11.3	11.7	12.1	12.5	12.9	13.2	13.6	14.0	14.4	14.8	15.2
8.3	8.6	8.9	9.3	9.6	9.9	10.2	10.5	10.9	11.2	11.5	11.8	12.2	12.5	12.8
5.8	6.0	6.2	6.4	6.7	6.9	7.1	7.3	7.6	7.8	8.0	8.2	8.5	8.7	8.9
10.0	10.4	10.7	11.1	11.5	11.9	12.3	12.7	13.1	13.5	13.9	14.2	14.6	15.0	15.4
6.9	7.2	7.5	7.7	8.0	8.3	8.5	8.8	9.1	9.4	9.6	9.9	10.2	10.4	10.7
7.8	8.1	8.4	8.7	9.0	9.3	9.6	9.9	10.2	10.5	10.8	11.1	11.4	11.7	12.0
5.7	5.9	6.1	6.3	6.5	6.8	7.0	7.2	7.4	7.6	7.9	8.1	8.3	8.5	8.7
10.7	11.1	11.5	11.9	12.3	12.8	13.2	13.6	14.0	14.4	14.8	15.2	15.7	16.1	16.5
7.6	7.9	8.2	8.5	8.8	9.1	9.4	9.7	10.0	10.3	10.6	10.9	11.2	11.4	11.7
7.9	8.2	8.5	8.8	9.2	9.5	9.8	10.1	10.4	10.7	11.0	11.3	11.6	11.9	12.2
6.8	7.1	7.3	7.6	7.8	8.1	8.4	8.6	8.9	9.2	9.4	9.7	10.0	10.2	10.5
7.9	8.2	8.5	8.8	9.1	9.5	9.8	10.1	10.4	10.7	11.0	11.3	11.6	11.9	12.2
9.1	9.4	9.8	10.1	10.5	10.8	11.2	11.5	11.9	12.2	12.6	12.9	13.3	13.6	14.0
10.2	10.6	11.0	11.4	11.8	12.2	12.6	13.0	13.4	13.8	14.2	14.6	14.9	15.3	15.7
1.4	1.5	1.5	1.6	1.6	1.7	1.7	1.8	1.8	1.9	1.9	2.0	2.1	2.1	2.2
6.7	7.0	7.3	7.5	7.8	8.1	8.3	8.6	8.8	9.1	9.4	9.6	9.9	10.2	10.4
5.4	5.6	5.8	6.0	6.2	6.4	6.7	6.9	7.1	7.3	7.5	7.7	7.9	8.1	8.3
2.7	2.8	2.9	3.0	3.1	3.2	3.3	3.4	3.5	3.6	3.7	3.9	4.0	4.1	4.2
11.2	11.6	12.1	12.5	12.9	13.4	13.8	14.2	14.7	15.1	15.5	16.0	16.4	16.8	17.3
4.6	4.8	4.9	5.1	5.3	5.5	5.7	5.8	6.0	6.2	6.4	6.5	6.7	6.9	7.1

CHAPTER 4
YOUR FIDGET LOG

WHAT'S THE BEST FIT BETWEEN ALL THE DIFFERENT WAYS you could move more and the details of your everyday activities? You are the expert on your own life. Only you know what's reasonable—what you're actually likely to do on a sustained basis. Or rather you will know after you begin to look at your day for chances to fidget.

Take advantage of this customized log to systematically ferret out fidget possibilities in just about everything you do. Remember that you won't have to burn too many calories at any one time. The idea is to make the cumulation of expended calories count for something.

Also remember that as long as you have either a leg or a hand free, the opportunity for movement is there. Almost anything can serve as a prop to push, pull, roll, squeeze, lift, whatever. Be especially on the lookout for things you can do that don't require much concentration. Make fidgeting a habit, part of the background noise of your life, part of you.

Using this log is simple: Keep your Fidget Log with you for the next week and write down every fidget activity you can devise at home, work, and other places. Try to come up with new ones each day of the first week. At the end of the week, go through your log and choose the most likely candidates for permanent inclusion in your daily fidgeting routine. After a month, edit the log according to what you found was really practical. That's all there is to it!

FIDGET LOG

Monday

Home:

Bedroom:

Kitchen:

Bathroom:

Living room:

Outdoors:

Work:

Tuesday

Home:

Bedroom:

Kitchen:

Bathroom:

Living room:

Outdoors:

Work:

Wednesday

Home:

Bedroom:

Kitchen:

Bathroom:

Living room:

Outdoors:

Work:

Thursday

Home:

    Bedroom:

    Kitchen:

    Bathroom:

    Living room:

Outdoors:

Work:

Friday

Home:

    Bedroom:

    Kitchen:

    Bathroom:

    Living room:

Outdoors:

Work:

Saturday

Home:

    Bedroom:

    Kitchen:

    Bathroom:

    Living room:

Outdoors:

Social Occasions:

FIDGET LOG

Sunday

Home:

  Bedroom:

  Kitchen:

  Bathroom:

  Living room:

Outdoors:

Work:

CHAPTER 5

DIET AND NUTRITION

IF YOU'VE EVER TAKEN B VITAMINS, YOU KNOW THAT they are made up of several components that need to be taken together. Those components work synergistically— they need each other, and it's in working as a group that they contribute to your well-being.

So it is with fidgeting, diet, and exercise. We have been emphasizing that fidgeting is an important factor in but nevertheless just a part of the routine that will put you where you want to be, weightwise. Fidgeting will work for you *only* if you do it in conjunction with eating a healthy diet and and engaging in a sensible, somewhat more vigorous exercise regimen.

You would be getting only part of the picture, part of the plan, if we did not spell out exactly what we meant by diet and exercise. We will begin with nutrition and dieting and the fad-dieting that most everyone has tried at least once. We assume that you've been there and done that and are now ready to settle down into the only kind of diet that works in the long run: a healthy one. We'll tell you what you need to know about body mass and body fat, and along the way, we'll take a look at your metabolism, the swing element that ties dieting to exercise.

THE SIMPLE FACT OF THE MATTER

It's a fact: The only way to control your weight and maintain your health is to combine regular exercise with a healthy diet. Most people aren't aware of this fact or choose to ignore it because at any given time, about 50 percent of Americans, from adolescents to seniors, are trying to lose weight or struggling to keep from putting on more weight. In their fight against fat, their diet holds center stage. It seems to be a matter of faith that the battle will be won or lost at the dinner table. They may add some exercise to the mix, but they regard it as secondary to their dietary scheme.

If you put the wrong kind of fuel in your car, it wouldn't matter how well the other systems were working, would it? The car couldn't possibly work at its best. It's the same with your body. You could fidget until you were blue in the face and it would get you nowhere in controlling your weight unless your diet was properly complementing your physical activities.

THE CALORIE IS KING

The food you eat contains a specific amount of potential energy, measured in calories. Some of that energy is burned off in the process of digestion, breathing, and other essential physical activities. Some of it is used to fuel whatever daily activities you engage in, everything from sitting up to shopping for groceries to making love to fixing a leaky faucet to jogging. Whatever doesn't get consumed ends up as body fat.

Your goal should be to find a combination of eating habits and exercise that enables you to comfortably balance the equation over the long run—to burn off at least

ONE OR THE OTHER

A report in the *Journal of the American Medical Association* stated that two-thirds of Americans who want to lose weight either watch their diet or engage in some form of exercise but do not do both. Among the 107,000 people who were studied who paid attention to their diet, many were diligently cutting back on fat while not being careful to limit calories from other sources, such as sugar.

as many calories as you take in to maintain weight, and to use up more calories as physical energy than come in with your food if your aim is to shed excess weight.

We're going to look at what goes into a sensible approach to "watching your weight." It starts with what you're shooting for in the first place, how you would like to look, and how you measure your progress toward that goal. Then we consider what's motivating you when you come to the table, and how you can modify a tendency to just eat and eat indiscriminately.

We will also lay out the basics of a healthy eating plan (*not* a diet). Finally, we will take a look at your metabolism, the bridge between diet and exercise. And along the way, you will see how fidgeting can work for you even when the subject is food.

YOUR SCALE IN THE SCHEME OF THINGS

We live in a digital dictatorship, gauging so many things in our life by the numbers. If weight control is an issue for you, then the digits on your scale may very well tell you whether you are going to allow yourself to feel good or bad about yourself today. That's not necessarily a great idea for at least two reasons.

JUST WHAT *IS* A CALORIE?

A calorie represents a unit of energy in the form of heat. Originally, it was defined as the amount of energy required at sea level to raise the temperature of a gram of water by one degree Celsius. However, when we use "calories" to describe the amount of energy in food, we really mean kilocalories, or units of a thousand calories. In other words, that slice of blueberry pie actually has 300,000 calories, equal to 300 kilocalories. We use the lower, more familiar number and as a kind of shorthand, refer to the unit as "calories."

And how do we know how many calories there are in a given amount of a specific kind of food, say, that slice of blueberry pie? We measure them with an instrument called a bomb calorimeter. The food is placed in a chamber surrounded by water and incinerated. The amount the temperature increases tells us the number of calories "burned" in the food.

First, keep in mind that what you want is to look better and feel better about yourself. That can never be measured in pounds per week. People are not going to judge you by your weight. They certainly will not evaluate you by how many pounds you did or did not take off since the last time they saw you.

Even if you've put on a few pounds, the clothes you're wearing, your demeanor, your hairstyle, the healthy glow that comes from eating the right food, even the expression on your face, are likely to have a lot more to do with the "way you look" than your exact weight. We know that you've probably heard this before, but it's still important to keep in mind because making a fetish of the numbers on the scale can become obsessive, causing you to lose your sense of proportion and making it harder for you to keep to any healthy eating plan.

Second, it's quite possible to be on track with your weight-control plan and not see much of a change in your weight just when you thought the numbers would become more favorable. For example, if you've been working out, you might have been increasing your muscle mass. So you could weigh about the same but still be in better shape and look better.

In fact, recently there has been a healthy trend away from relying solely on pounds in evaluating one's physical condition. The newer focus is on what *constitutes* your weight—how much of it is fat and how much is leaner tissue such as muscle. For purposes of health, doctors and those who scientifically study exercise are paying more attention to exactly where that body fat tends to be stored.

TIP ON FEELING BETTER ABOUT YOUR WEIGH-IN

On those days when you get on the scale, you can reduce your anxiety through a little last-minute exercise. Sure, it's too late to swim another lap, sneak in another mile of jogging, or fifteen more minutes of pedaling or walking. But you can easily do a few fidgeting routines right up to the moment you set foot on the scale. In fact, one of the routines involves the scale itself. Try these (assuming your scale is in the bathroom):

- Punch out the shower curtain. (Seriously.) Do it for three minutes and if you weigh 132 pounds, you will burn about 17 calories.

- Pick up a bottle in each hand (shampoo, conditioner, whatever you see) and move each hand, one at a time, straight out from your body and then back. If you weigh 137 pounds, three minutes of this will use up about 11 calories.

- Now hold those bottles with your arms straight down at your sides. Swing your left arm forward while you swing the right one back behind you. Reverse, swinging the right forward and the left back. Do it for five minutes and you will burn 18.5 calories.

YOUR BODY MASS

There's more to you than can be measured in pounds. You may have heard of the Body Mass Index, or BMI, a measurement that looks at your weight relative to your height. This figure is calculated by plugging your weight and height into a formula—it's your weight in pounds multiplied by your height in inches squared, with the result multiplied by 703. (You can look up your BMI on a chart in the back of this book, so you don't have to worry about the math.) The result is expressed in a two-digit number, usually ranging from the high teens to the thirties. This measurement works for men and women over the age of eighteen, without regard to one's frame. It is not accurate for athletes who have considerable muscle mass, for pregnant women, or for sedentary or frail older people.

For example, if you are five feet four and weigh 115 pounds, your BMI is 19.8, which puts you in the "healthy" category. You still might not be satisfied with how you look, but then you would be shedding pounds for purely cosmetic reasons. The same would hold true for someone who was six feet two and weighed 170 pounds, producing a BMI of 21.9. A BMI over 25 is considered overweight; a BMI in excess of 30 suggests obesity.

When it comes to fat, it's not just what you've got but also where it's at. You are considered healthier, at least in terms of your prospective longevity, if the fat is concentrated in your lower body, rather than around your abdomen—if you resemble a pear rather than an apple. In general, according to the National Institutes of Health, a woman should have a waist size less than thirty-five inches, while men should come in at below forty inches.

What does all of this mean to you? It means that you need to keep some perspective on the very concept of

IT PAYS TO REDUCE YOUR BMI

According to a study published in the October 1999 *Journal of the American Medical Association,* lowering your BMI by 10 percent, on average, will reduce your lifetime medical costs by $2,200 to $5,300. On a national scale, we also pay for calories run amok. Graham Colditz of the Harvard School of Public Health and Anne Wolf of the University of Virginia wrote that in 1995, excess body fat cost Americans almost $100 billion in lost work time due to illness, decreased productivity, and trips to the doctor.

"weight." What's really important is to avoid being "over-fat," not overweight. Even if you appear thin, you could still be overfat, with fat stored in the abdominal area where you can see it as folds in your skin. And a big-framed, heavily muscled athlete, like many of the professional football players we have worked with, can be conventionally overweight while coming in well under the level of body fat that would make him overfat. So although such an athlete may be "overweight," there is no real need for weight loss.

If your BMI suggests that you have a serious problem, it would probably be worth your while to get a more complete health-risk analysis by your health-care professional.

Ideally, men should have 12 to 18 percent body fat and women, 21 to 28 percent. You can get a reasonably accurate determination of your body's fat content at a medical center or even at your local Y. A more exact measurement is obtained by taking a person's weight underwater. People with higher body fat will weigh less underwater with respect to their weight out of water because, ironically, lean tissue, primarily muscle mass, weighs more than body fat. Since this is not a very convenient method, more often body fat is measured by placing a caliper on a fold of skin, or it's done electronically.

EATING: HOW DO YOU *FEEL* ABOUT IT?

Body fat is a potential problem that you can deal with at its source: your eating habits. Why not head it off *before* it becomes an issue in you life?

If we were all perfectly rational, we wouldn't have to worry about the food we eat. We would eat what was good for us, and only as much as we needed. But we know very few people who fit that description.

If you're a parent or have ever spent much time with an infant, you have probably noticed what kind of a schedule babies have when it comes to eating. They eat when they're hungry. It's that simple. When they're full, they stop. In their world, there's a certain amount of "common sense" when it comes to food.

But babies become children who eat in time slots. Food takes on multiple meanings, often becoming a function of mood. Children learn to eat or not to eat out of emotional need, using food as a comfort to soothe themselves when they feel distressed. Sometimes dinner becomes a weapon in a tug-of-war with a parent over issues unrelated to food. Or eating can even become an antidote to boredom or loneliness.

By the time they are adults, eating is often caught up in a highly charged drama. They may eat too much and the wrong things for reasons that have little to do with hunger.

For example, every time Sid Stoneman, a customer relations specialist with a large retail chain, finds that he's stuffing himself at the dinner table, he has a flashback of the sumptuous holiday meals his mother prepared when he was a kid. But those memories come with a price. He can still hear her complain of "slaving" in the kitchen to put that feast on the table, the implication being that he should show his gratitude by cleaning his plate. And so he does. In fact, at home he even pulls his guests into this reenactment of a childhood drama, insisting that they eat beyond their capacity as well, to show that they really appreciate the meal.

We don't generate all of our irrational eating habits by ourselves. Outside the home, the world is a minefield of temptation. If it isn't that heavenly restaurant dessert that gets you, it's the candy counter at the movies. Along with the pure temptation comes social pressure. It's harder to resist when everyone else is giving in. Everyone around you is munching, why not you?

Even your job can put temptation in your way. Loretta Philips, an administrative assistant in the orthopedic department of a large medical center, had been pretty good at watching the calories. But what constantly tripped her up were the office celebrations for birthdays, promotions, and retirements. Between all these events, there always seemed to be a perpetually filled candy dish on one of the filing cabinets or irresistible slices of chocolate cake with icing on one of the desks just as you came in the door. Loretta finally managed to get some control over her cravings by burying herself in her work on such occasions or allowing herself only a taste of the cake, but it wasn't easy.

Some people also snack destructively between meals— candy, pastry, potato chips, you name it—as a reward for making it through a rough day at the office or as a consolation for not doing so. Work is often tough enough on one's nerves and stamina; it shouldn't have to threaten the waistline as well!

DIETING: NOT ONLY IS IT IRRATIONAL, BUT IT DOESN'T WORK

It doesn't help to compound our irrational eating styles with well-meaning but equally irrational countermeasures aimed at pushing back weight gain. But that's what most people do when they go on a diet—any diet.

Between compulsion and temptation, we are primed for anything that we think might protect us from overeating and eating foods we "shouldn't." We spend a fortune on diet books and diet programs, health club membership fees, home exercise equipment, and workout clothing. It's a measure of our desperation in our war against fat that almost any new fad diet can have its day—some pretty outrageous and sometimes dangerous ones holding the spotlight for months or even years.

The public appetite for fad diets, especially, seems to be voracious and incapable of being fully satisfied. One year, cabbage is king; the next year, grapefruit is in. Perhaps there's something wonderful about the sound of the word "protein," because millions of people are willing to see protein diets as the authentic key to being slim. Its popularity may even stem from the belief—current as recently as a generation or two ago—that a high-protein diet promotes good health. It does echo the once-held notion that a meat dinner every night, for those who could afford it, was the right way to feed a family.

High-protein diets, in particular, can play havoc with nutrition and what we know about food and the way our

WEIGHT WATCHING

Dieting has almost been a national custom since World War I, when counting calories was emphasized by the government as an efficient way of maintaining sufficient food supplies and avoiding shortages, and the 1920s, when the penny scale first came into widespread public use. By 1970, we had Weight Watchers, and the sale of appetite-suppressant pills was hitting $2 billion a year. Now, according to the Mayo Clinic, we spend over $33 billion a year on products and services geared to helping us lose weight, but the number of overweight adults in this country continues to grow at the rate of about 1 percent a year.

bodies use it. To people who believe in them, diets high in protein were the original, natural, healthy diets, what our ancestors ate before civilization misled us. Proponents suggest that excessive carbohydrates somehow dangerously boost our insulin levels. Therefore the way to get rid of excess weight is to load up on protein while cutting carbohydrate consumption.

It is certainly possible to overdo the carbohydrates in your diet, especially the simple ones such as sugar, and even some of the more complex ones such as bread and pasta. But being on a low-carbohydrate diet for too long is itself harmful. What they're telling you is to increase the amount of fat in your diet—that's what often comes along with food high in protein—while de-emphasizing fruits and vegetables. From what you already know about over-consumption of fat and the importance of the vitamins and minerals we get from fruits and vegetables, how much sense can that make? Not much.

A healthy diet contains less than 30 percent fat, 15 percent or less of protein, and 55 to 60 percent carbohydrates. There shouldn't be any sharp deviation from this formula—it's pretty much that simple for most of us.

LIVING OFF THE FAT OF THE LAND

Somewhere around 1998, the manager of Gallagher's Steak House in New York City, which displays slabs of beef in its window, noticed a trend among diners. "People are coming in, and they're just eating steak. They're not eating potatoes or bread," he said in amazement. "They eat prime beef steaks and creamed spinach, and insist they're on a diet. It blows me away." If you also share the outlook that the only thing you have to fear in a cheeseburger is the bun, the cholesterol in your blood could blow you away, too.

There are some regimens that promise the shedding of excess pounds if only we will follow the guru of the moment. Or just give a particular diet five days a week and it will give us a "miracle." (We're waiting for the book authored by some doctor that will claim that you can achieve complete nutrition and lose or maintain weight by consuming only apple pie and tequila!)

More than anything else, the popularity of fad diets demonstrates our faith in the power of dieting itself. This hunger to find the one angle we've missed so far is also a clear measure of our desperation to overcome our recognition that ultimately *most gimmick diets, those emphasizing only one food, usually fail.*

Of course, proponents of fad diets can always produce people for whom they have worked—at least in the short run. You may even know someone who's had that experience. There's nothing like a "before and after" comparison to get people to sit up and take notice and maybe be willing to try it themselves.

But what you see is not always what you get. High-protein diets, for example, can give you a quick weight loss because they promote the excretion of water—like a sponge being wrung out—and the consumption of only a few calories, which is also the reason why you're likely to regain the weight as soon as you give up on the diet. And giving up is what most people finally do when the novelty wears off and the diet becomes, as Jennifer K. Nelson, a clinical dietician at the Mayo Clinic put it, "a ball and chain."

What do all of these diets have in common? They are variations on the quick fix. If you've gone down this path yourself, you know how likely it is that somewhere along the line you will put that weight back on. You also know the sense of deprivation that can pervade your life while you're on such a diet. As *New York Times* personal health columnist Jane Brody, who has given up dieting altogether, recalled, "Dieting made me super-conscious of food. It also caused me to suffer from *deprivation syndrome.* After denying myself food, I would binge."

In fact, not only is dieting as we usually do it a psychological formula for failure, but it can even stack the cards against you, especially if you try to take too much weight off too quickly. Such a regimen can lower your metabolism, the rate at which you convert food to energy. It can cause you to store more of the food in the form of fat rather than dissipate the calories as heat. Then look what you've got: a body that's become more efficient at storing fat. Now any exercise you do is less productive. This is definitely not progress.

You're better off forgetting about any specialized diet unless it's been prescribed by your doctor to counter some specific health problem. Trying somehow to sculpt your diet by juggling protein, carbohydrates, and any other basic component of it with the hope that you've found the key to it all is as useful as trying to use exercise for spot weight-reduction: It simply won't work.

THAT DIET STATE OF MIND

Diet often enough and you may develop a certain obsessive mind-set that could result in self-defeating behavior. Canadian researchers told dieters in an experiment that they had each put on five pounds. Consequently they felt bad about their efforts to lose weight, let their guard drop, and compensated for their bad feelings by overeating. Subjects in the experiment who were not dieting, but also told that they had gained five pounds, did not change their eating habits.

Nor does slashing your calorie intake with abandon bring good results. Never go to extremes with a reduction in calories that flirts with starvation. Aside from the obvious health risks, it doesn't work either, except for giving you a temporary hollow-cheeked look. Not eating enough is unhealthy and just slows your metabolism so that you become less efficient in burning calories. When you begin to eat more, as inevitably you will, the weight could come back with a vengeance.

WHY AND WHEN TO PUT A NEW EATING PLAN INTO EFFECT

Here's what we suggest: Throw away the diet books, the audiocassettes, and the video tapes with the pronouncements from diet gurus; keep only the calorie charts and the booklets you can get free from the Department of Agriculture (www.usda.gov) and information from other reliable sources about the components of a healthy diet. What you need is not to go *on* a diet, but rather to *eat* a variety of good foods. If you exercise and your basic approach to eating is in good shape, eventually you will be, too.

That's worth repeating: Eating the right food is also the best way to have your diet contribute its share to your overall weight control program. You will find that if you concentrate on the right food and increase your exercise, the calories will start to take care of themselves.

How do you get started? First, it's not a good idea to change your eating habits while chaos rules. If you're under pressure because you have a project deadline looming, or if you're going to be traveling in the immediate future, wait until a more tranquil or stable time to really get into it. Also, contrary to what many people think, the time to start getting control of what happens at the dinner table is not when you're down in the dumps and figure that a quick weight loss will pull you out of it.

A healthy eating plan is something you should look forward to, a kind of empowerment that puts you at the steering wheel of your own life. That's why the decision to change in this way should be yours. Letting someone else's agenda suggest how you should govern the most basic parts of your life is surely a recipe for failure. Don't do it because someone else wants you to, whether that's a friend, spouse, or lover. First decide that it's what *you* want to do, because without self-motivation, it won't work. It has to be your plan, tailored to your needs and tastes.

When you do decide that you're ready, be sure to have realistic expectations. The last thing in the world you want is to be lured into one of those yo-yo situations where your weight goes up and down. You need to be on a more even keel.

This important point can't be emphasized too much: It's unreasonable to think that you can lose more than two pounds a week over time and keep it off. The rush that a quick loss will give you will soon be forgotten when the weight comes creeping back—and the chances are good that it will.

EAT RIGHT, EAT IN MODERATION

So what should guide you when you decide that you want to eat better? When it comes to working off or warding off weight by what you do at the dinner table, *the only approach that really makes sense, that works in the long run, is to eat more of the fruits, vegetables, and whole grains that research has shown to be at the heart of a healthy diet, and less of the fatty, sugary, starchy foods that unfortunately predominate in the American diet.*

As far as quantity goes, here's an easy mnemonic device to remind yourself not to pile it on the plate: *To keep your sense of proportion, keep your eye on the portion.* Read the labels on all prepared and packaged foods you buy and just remember that you're eating only for one.

Eating in moderation also means not inducing a sense of deprivation. You will feel better if instead of cutting out completely foods that you enjoy, you cut back. Unless your diet rules out certain foods entirely because of a medical condition, eating almost anything once in a while should not hurt you. That means a slice of pizza, a sirloin steak, or even a banana split. You will find that if you "give in" in this small way, you won't feel as if you are suffering and you'll find it easier to stay in control of your "cravings."

PROACTIVE EATING

How can you eat moderate-sized portions without having your plate look like someone has already gotten to it ahead of you? Well, you could use a smaller plate, according to health columnist Jane Brody, who follows her own advice. She also mixes several different kinds of foods on the plate, letting variety add an extra pleasure.

IT DOESN'T TAKE MUCH

Eating moderately by cutting back instead of cutting out isn't as hard as it sounds. You can do it! For example, eliminating 50 empty calories a day from your diet will result in a five-pound weight loss over the course of a year. You won't miss those calories too much. There's about that much in

A tablespoon of honey: 60 calories

Three packaged sugar cubes: 45

One slice of Arnold Brick Oven White Bread: 70

On the other hand, it doesn't take much to throw your diet out of kilter. Let's say, for example, that you have a craving for roasted peanuts. If you add just two ounces a day of this treat to a diet that is already in balance—that is, you're working off as many calories as you're taking in—you will gain in excess of seven pounds in the course of a single year!

Eating earlier in the day also helps. It works because the calories you pick up are more likely to be burned off than to end up as fat you-know-where. Also helpful is to eat more often but to have smaller meals. A large meal gets your digestive system to work overtime. You end up digesting food faster and being hungry sooner, as well. And by all means, try to eat only when you're truly hungry (remember the wisdom of babies!).

Don't let food happen to you. If you take control of your eating habits, you can deny those extra calories a role in your life without suffering from self-denial in the process. The trick is to use your whole head, your brain as well as your mouth, in choosing what goes into you and what doesn't. Here are some more practical things you can do to stay on top of the calories so that they don't end up on top of you:

- Eat more at breakfast so that you take in a greater percentage of your total calories earlier in the day, when your body is better at burning off the excess.

- Have your dessert of the day with lunch, not dinner. More of it will get converted into energy rather than into more of you because you'll burn more energy as the day goes on.

- What's your idea of a treat for guests? As many people like popcorn as crave ice cream, and popcorn makes less of a mess. Or you could substitute fruit sorbet for the ice cream and dress it up with a decorative wafer. Conversely, when you're going to be the guest, come prepared: Eat a little something before you go, so you're not overwhelmed by whatever your host has waiting for you.

- When temptation is put in your way (did we hear someone say "buffet"?), don't deny yourself completely, but make whatever you take a "singular sensation," as they say on Broadway. Take one piece or one slice. You will feel better about yourself and still not feel left out of the fun.

Any or all of these techniques may help you to stay with good eating habits and not discard them, as dieters often do with their regimens. Persistence is important because even with the best combination of physical activities and good diet, any initial loss of weight is likely to be from losing water and carbohydrates. Body fat takes longer to disappear.

Snacking, usually thought of as a source of weight gain, can be employed as a means of weight control. Your body will crave at least some fuel every three to four hours, and if you can eat small quantities of food that will both provide energy and fill you up so you don't go off the deep end between meals, you will be ahead of the game.

Grain-based snacks fill this bill very well—fat-free rice cakes, whole wheat bread sticks, graham crackers, and pretzels (try one dipped in salsa!) are all fine. You won't go wrong either with a piece of fresh fruit, dried fruit such as papaya or apricot (if fresh fruit is too messy), a carrot stick, or a celery stalk. You can pack them in your briefcase or handbag, stash a snack at your desk, and, of course, when you're home, make sure that the makings of a snack are always available in the cupboard and refrigerator.

EATING OUT

Just as modern technology has made our lives easier but softer, so greater access to restaurant meals has increased our waistlines at the same time that it has taken more work out of daily living. Do you usually serve yourself portions as large as you get when you eat out? Probably not. But here's where you can put technology in the service of watching your weight. Ask for a doggy bag and *use* that microwave oven on which you spent almost $200. Or you could share an entrée with your dinner companion, or not order any entrée and instead have just an appetizer and a salad.

If you're dining at a full-service restaurant, ask for some carrot sticks or celery stalks if they're available. That will keep your hands occupied and away from the bread and butter and you will also be getting some fiber into you before you're tempted to start picking out some rich appetizer. Of course, you could simply ask the waiter to remove the bread—out of sight, out of mouth.

Anyplace where there are hors d'oeuvres is a potential danger zone. For example, at weddings, they may bring them around on a tray and you will suddenly find them right under your nose. That's a good time for a little creative fidgeting—anything to keep your hands busy. You could keep some coins in your pocket to manipulate, or even "nurse" a bread stick for half an hour while you fiddle with it. (There's the beauty of the fidget factor: You couldn't occupy yourself with push-ups at a wedding!) You could also take the approach of a tray of goodies as your signal to make the rounds from table to table or, if there's music, to get up and dance.

If you still have trouble eating less and choosing the right foods, you could put to use the findings of psychologists in a study at Iowa State University. They discovered that people who were having that kind of problem did better if there was a mirror that reflected what went on the dinner table. Either people were catching themselves in the act of piling it on their plates, or the thought of seeing themselves overeating acted as a deterrent.

THINK POSITIVELY

Do you ever just throw up your arms in surrender and ascribe your weight problems to genes? Sure, genetic inheritance affects our tendency to have bodies that look a certain way. But your parents and more distant ancestors probably play less of a role than you might think. If heredity is all that important, why did the biggest gain in what the average American weighs come between 1980 and 1994? As Dr. William H. Dietz, director of the Division of Nutrition and Physical Activity at the Centers for Disease Control and Prevention, observed, during that period "the genes did not change substantially."

YOU MAY NOT WANT TO KNOW THIS

A McDonald's Quarter Pounder with Cheese has 520 calories and 29 grams of fat. Since 1 gram of fat equals 9 calories, that's 29 x 9 = 261 calories, or 50 percent of the quarter pounder! You might as well pour an ounce of pure oil into your arteries. A tuna salad sandwich at one of the Subway sandwich franchise stores is even worse, socking you with 522 calories and 33 grams of fat. But sometimes you're rushed and only fast food is available. At those times, practice self-defense. Choose dishes without cheese or mayonnaise (mustard is fine). Look for lean meat such as turkey. And stay away from fried foods.

At full-service restaurants, watch out for the drink before dinner that not only adds mostly empty calories but also dulls your judgment just before you see the menu. Start with a salad to keep your mouth busy, your stomach engaged, and your hands away from the breadbasket. Grilled entrées minimize fat. If you really want something that you know is not for the best, order a small portion. And dessert? Share, unless it's your birthday or anniversary.

This is good news. It means that it's within your power to have a substantial effect on the way you look and feel by altering your behavior. Don't approach this task as if it were going to be torture. You're not going to go on a diet; rather, you're going to be switching to eating healthier food. Yes, you should count calories, and probably keep your diet under 2,500 calories a day—the specific amount depending on gender, size, and level of physical activity—that's an essential part of eating in moderation. But there's a lot you can do within those limits. There's a world of taste, variety, and pleasure in foods that are good for you, as well.

Keep in mind that you are aiming at a good eating style, which is even more important than if you came in under your calorie quota for any given day. Let your self-esteem be tied to your success in eating the right foods.

Measure your accomplishment not against the occasional backsliding but rather in the context of good foods you didn't eat before but that are now part of your diet, supplanting empty calories with nutritionally filled ones. Remind yourself that what you are doing is not aimed at quick weight loss but rather at keeping off the pounds and shedding fat in the long term.

Don't hold yourself to impossibly high standards. That means not being conned into thinking you have to look like those size 6 female models or the male models who seem constitutionally incapable of having more than a size 30 waist. Your gradual, even modest weight loss will do what you want it to do, making you look better and reducing the danger to your health that comes with high blood pressure and high cholesterol.

Eating the right amount of good food may sound difficult, but you have been well armed to accomplish this mission. There are easily available charts telling you how many calories there are in just about any kind of food you are likely to eat. And federal law requires that any prepared or packaged food that you buy have a label detailing its nutritional content.

Now let's deal with the components of your diet that you need to keep in mind in planning what you want to eat.

YOUR BODY IN THE BALANCE

It's fitting that the U.S. Department of Agriculture uses a food pyramid to visually represent the dishes that should go into your diet. It tells us that a balanced diet begins with a solid foundation, on which everything else rests. For a healthy diet, that foundation is built on bread, cereal,

LOOK UP THE NUMBERS

It's a good idea to keep handy a chart that will give you the caloric value of a wide variety of foods. But if you don't have one or are on the computer and want to quickly check the calorie content of a dish, try the calorie counter at

www.caloriecontrol.org/.

pasta, and rice—the familiar carbohydrates. On top of them come fruits and vegetables; above them are the protein-rich dairy products, meat, poultry, eggs; and at the pinnacle, situated at the point so that you get the point, are the foods that are best used sparingly—oils, fats, and sweets.

The idea is to chose most of your calories from the base of the pyramid, to work from the bottom up, eating more sparingly those foods that are set above. But *don't confuse calories with quantity.* Small quantities of the carbohydrates at the bottom of the pyramid will provide you with the all the calories you need. Bread, cereal, pasta, and rice have adequate calories per unit volume of food, so your portions of these dishes should be on the smaller side, while vegetables and fruits, which have relatively few calories, should fill more of your plate, with dairy and meat components used in modest amounts to provide enough protein and other necessary vitamins and minerals in your diet.

Vegetables and fruits are nature's health bargain. From them you can obtain the vitamins, minerals, fiber, and other substances you need for good health, while not piling on the calories. They also fill you up the way fat-laden dishes cannot, so you're less likely to be set up for eating what you shouldn't before your next meal. A good diet

START BURNING CALORIES WHILE YOU'RE COOKING

Most nutritionists will tell you that cooking a meal from raw ingredients (providing that those ingredients are healthy ones) is always better than using prepared foods. But how often do you hear anyone discuss the physical fitness bonus that comes with cooking? When you cook your own food, you're burning calories in a physical activity while you're preparing to add calories from eating. In fact, you can burn 200 calories while cooking for about an hour, as many as you would burn paddling a canoe at a slow pace—enough to offset the amount you would take in eating a potato stuffed with bacon and cheese.

---

would include at least two servings of fruit and five of vegetables every day. You can get much-needed calcium with several servings of low-fat dairy foods.

The opposite of the bargain foods are the empty foods, good only for a little quick energy. They contain mostly sugar, which pays off in more calories but nothing good to go along with it. (Well, okay, they can taste great in the form of desserts. But do you really want to pay the caloric price, not to mention the danger from their fat content?)

The sugar content of the American diet—in addition to the naturally occurring sugar content of foods, such as fruit—has been increasing at an unhealthy rate. In 1986, sugar consumption was at 127 pounds per person per year. By 1994, it had hit 144 and was at 156 pounds in 1998.

Americans average nineteen to twenty teaspoons of sugar a day, mostly in their coffee, desserts, and prepared foods, often to compensate for "reduced fat." The sugar in some of these foods could sneak right by you. An example is fruit yogurt, eight ounces of which will give you

DIET MEETS EXERCISE

There's another benefit from drinking water. If you consume eight glasses a day and make sure you have to get up to get each one of them, that's a pretty decent amount of calorie-consuming movement. Not to mention the several extra trips to the bathroom that greater consumption of water will necessitate. Altogether you will burn about an extra 10 to 20 calories a day because of it.

seven teaspoons of sugar that you may not have been counting on.

Yes, fruit sugar and table sugar deliver the same amount of calories. But just remember that fruit sugar is part of a package deal that delivers other nutrients, while in addition to a little energy, table sugar offers ... well, tooth decay. And fruit is high in fiber and is filling, helping to curb your appetite, while something like candy leaves you grabbing for more. For example, a medium-sized orange will give you about 65 calories and satisfy your hunger. Five gumdrops will deliver about the same number of calories, but do you think you're really going to stop there?

But what about the energy that sugar supplies? Having a sugary treat and then burning it off by immediately engaging in some physical activity won't hurt. But if you're feeling tired, in fact, what you may need is not sugar but water. You can be dehydrated and barely feel thirsty, but what you *will* feel is tired. Try to drink at least eight glasses of water a day.

CARBOHYDRATES

There are three basic food elements that must be in your diet because your body needs them to function optimally. They are the only substances your body can burn to convert into energy: carbohydrates, protein, and fat. They appear in varying amounts in all the food in your diet, ranging from merely a trace of fat in most vegetables to a good deal of protein in meat and eggs. If your diet has a sensible mix of foods from the food pyramid, these elements will be in balance, and the vitamins and minerals you also need will be there in sufficient quantities to maintain your health.

The problem is that most Americans don't achieve that balance. Even many people who think they are diligently eating a balanced diet often fall short of it by not paying enough attention to the size of their portions. That's when the extra calories sneak in.

That's especially true of the carbohydrates, which should constitute about 60 percent of your total food intake during the day. We've already dealt with simple carbohydrates, which are represented in your diet by sugar and other sweeteners; they have little nutritional value. Complex carbohydrates, such as fruits, vegetables, pasta, bread, and cereals contain fiber, a useful ingredient for anyone trying to control his or her weight because it leaves you feeling full longer and thus less likely to eat what you shouldn't. Making sure that each meal is higher in fiber means you're less likely to overeat at that meal. Also, diets high in fiber have been shown to lower the risk of cancers of the stomach, colon, and rectum.

The complex carbohydrates are also excellent sources of long-term, slow-burning energy that stores in your muscles. That's why marathon runners often load up on pasta the night before a big race.

But even among the complex carbohydrates, things aren't so simple. Some complex carbohydrates, such as white rice and white bread, are low in other nutrients and

RICE CAKES VS. CHOCOLATE CHIP COOKIES

Which is the better snack? It's not as obvious as you may think: It depends on what's on the label. For example, we recently picked up some naturally flavored apple-cinnamon rice cakes at a local health food store. A serving was one cake, which provided 80 calories, 0.5 grams of fat, and less than 1 gram of fiber. Compare that to fat-free chocolate chip cookies from the same store made with whole-wheat flour and nonfat milk. The three small cookies that made for one serving provided 100 calories, no fat, and 3 grams of fiber. The fiber was the clincher. In fact, you could pop just one of these bite-sized treats in your mouth and be satisfied. What you'd eat would total just 33 calories, no fat, some nutrition, and more than a gram of fiber (you should try to consume 25 to 30 grams of fiber a day). As for which tastes better . . . that's your call!

fiber compared to other complex carbohydrates. As with all your food purchases, reading the labels on these and other products will help to keep you on track.

There's another problem you may run into with carbohydrates. Alice Stanton discovered it only after years of having a big dish of pasta at least three times a week. Alice, a paralegal living in Boston, simply could not cut down on the size of her portions, or even on the number of times each week she ate pasta. She felt a strange kind of deprivation each time she tried to limit this dish.

For many people, carbohydrates are a "mood food." Dishes like spaghetti boost the amount of serotonin in the brain. That can have a calming, even slightly tranquilizing effect—often just what you might think you need after a tough day at the office. Alice finally got this problem under control by having a pretzel as a late-afternoon snack, which gave her some needed carbohydrates and made that pasta in the evening a little easier to turn away from completely or, as on some nights, to have as a small side dish to a vegetarian dinner.

PROTEIN

Poultry, meat, dairy products, beans, and nuts are the main sources of dietary protein. You need the amino acids in protein because they are your body's building blocks. You use them to make muscle and build and replenish tissue throughout your body. The body doesn't store this vital substance, so you should have some every day. (But eat too much of it and your body *will* store it—as fat!) We need 0.8 grams of protein a day for every 2.2 pounds of body weight. A woman over the age of twenty-five weighing about 130 pounds requires 45 to 50 grams a day, and a man over twenty-five weighing about 175 pounds would need approximately 60 to 65 grams. Thirty grams is equivalent to just over an ounce of protein.

Despite what you might have heard when you were a child, you definitely *can* get too much protein. The most obvious reason is that if you go over these numbers, or the equivalent intake for your age and weight, you are almost certainly eating too much fat, because the highest amount of protein is to be found in animal products, which also have the greatest fat content. Overdoing it with proteins also puts a strain on your kidneys and makes it harder to get your metabolism to work as efficiently to burn calories.

The advantage of animal products is that they contain all the amino acids—the building blocks of protein—your body needs, and they are thus known as "complete" proteins. The solution to getting all the amino acids you need but not overdosing on fat involves going easy on proteins, eating small portions and perhaps using meat just to flavor dishes, or, if you're a vegetarian, using a combination of food that will give you all the amino acids you need. The two most popular combinations are soup and bread and rice and beans, two of the world's most popular dishes. Another solution is to eat six to seven ounces of fish per week, such as tuna, sardines, or salmon—which are high in the kinds of fats that actually help to reduce cholesterol and increase HDL, the "good" cholesterol—beefing up your fish consumption reduces the risk of heart disease.

EATING VS. EXERCISE

Always keep in mind that you can lop off calories by what you *do*, as well as by what you *don't* do. Here's a trade-off comparison between some dishes you can skip and some low-level, nonsweat exercise and fidgeting you can do:

- A cup of rice pudding: 33 calories
- A hard roll and a pat of butter: 200
- A three-ounce hamburger from lean ground beef: 230
- Strolling for thirty minutes at two miles an hour: 100
- Playing the guitar for thirty minutes: 110
- Horsing around with the kids for thirty minutes: 150
- Rolling a rubber ball round and round under your foot for ten minutes while reading the newspaper: 26
- While in the kitchen preparing a meal, during those periods when you're watching, waiting, and occasionally stirring, pick up a can of soup in each hand and lift one straight up in the air, then the other. Keep alternating for ten minutes to expend 30 calories

FAT DOESN'T CARRY ITS WEIGHT IN YOUR WEIGHT-CONTROL PLAN

You can't live without fat, but then you can't live without arsenic, either. You need some fat in your diet for several reasons. Fat provides energy, and some vitamins require the presence of fat to be assimilated. You need fat to manufacture hormones. Fat also adds flavor to food and in reasonable quantities, it would not be the problem it's been made out to be.

But the typical American diet includes way too much of this potentially dangerous substance. Between fast-food double cheeseburgers, French fries, bacon-and-egg breakfasts, Danish, doughnuts, and rich sauces and gravy at dinnertime, we are constantly flirting with danger. Fat is also a problem because it's often lurking in large quantities, mixed with other things, and is therefore not so obvious. For example, a tablespoon of salad dressing can contain fourteen grams of fat!

Fat works against your efforts to control your weight, since it is the most concentrated fuel. A gram of fat contains slightly more than twice the number of calories as one gram of protein or sugar!

According to the book *Fitness without Exercise* (Warner Books, 1990), by Bryant A. Stamford and Porter Shimer, eating fatty foods also prevents your metabolism from working as your ally. When you eat nonfatty foods, your body has to convert more of the food into energy just to metabolize it and store it as body fat than it does if it's fat that's being digested. For example, you have to burn only about 5 calories to turn 100 calories of the fat from French fries or a Big Mac into fat that is now part of you. But if that 100 calories comes from pasta or whole grains, you will consume 30 calories before that rigatoni or whole wheat bread is fat tissue in your body.

Not only does the process of digesting fat cheat you of the greater number of calories that you could be burning if you were eating nonfatty foods, but fat itself has more calories per unit volume than other foods. Here are some basic numbers to think about the next time you're in the mood for a burger and a Bud:

- There are 9 calories in every gram of fat.
- There are 7 calories in every gram of alcohol.
- There are 4 calories each in every gram of protein and carbohydrates.

FAT: THE HIDDEN DANGER

You've heard this before, but it's worth repeating: If you eat too much fat, particularly the wrong kinds of it, your arteries can become clogged with fatty deposits, eventually leading to a heart attack or a stroke. This process goes on silently over the years, and you may have no warning before heart disease becomes evident.

The main culprit in this drama seems to be cholesterol. Your cholesterol should measure below 200 milligrams per 100 milliliters of blood. The typical middle-aged American has a cholesterol level of about 230. If that doesn't sound too bad, consider this: Men with a cholesterol reading of 260 are three times as likely to have a heart attack as those whose cholesterol is 195.

But don't be misled by claims on food packages of "low cholesterol" or "no cholesterol." After infancy, your body manufactures all the cholesterol you need, so clearly you do not want to take in any extra in your diet if you can avoid it.

EXERCISE AND YOUR CHOLESTEROL

Here's another area where exercise can work with your diet plan. But this time the relationship between exercise and diet is direct. Cholesterol needs help to circulate in your body—to get to your artery walls where it forms a substance called plaque that can block the flow of blood. A substance called low-density lipoproteins, or LDL, a component of cholesterol, provides this transport system for cholesterol. Eating too much food containing saturated fats promotes the production of LDL by your liver, and results in more cholesterol being deposited in your arteries.

On the other hand, high-density lipoproteins, or HDL, gather excess cholesterol in your blood and transport it to your liver, which gets rid of it. Regular aerobic and strengthening exercise training increases your body's level of HDL, decreasing your body's total cholesterol.

The biggest source of excess cholesterol in your blood is actually saturated fat, which your body converts into cholesterol. Potentially, it's the wrong kind of fat that can kill.

Here are some of the most common sources of saturated fat in our diets:

Butter
Whole milk
Cheese
Egg yolks
Luncheon meats
Franks, hamburgers, bacon, and marbled red meat
Pastry
Sauces and gravy
Ice cream
Chocolate (ouch!)
Coconut and palm oils

As you can see when you consult a food label, there are several kinds of fats. The most common have names that refer to their molecular structure: saturated, polyunsaturated, and monounsaturated. But you don't need an electron microscope to tell them apart. At room temperature, saturated fats (butter, for example) are solid; monounsaturated (olive oil), thick liquids; and polyunsaturated (corn and soybean oils), liquid. The mono- and polyunsaturated fats help your body to control cholesterol and in moderate quantities, are good to have in your diet. When you look at a food label, look for a ratio of at least two to one in favor of the mono- and unsaturated fats with respect to saturated fat.

Some food, such as margarine, which is not made from saturated fat, is solid at room temperature. Margarine, for example, is hydrogenated—made solid—for convenience, so you can spread it. Such fats are not good for you, and you should beware of them as you are of saturated fat. If fat has been partially hydrogenated—the case in many kinds of margarine—it's okay if there is also plenty of polyunsaturated fat in the product.

Another problematic fat is the trans fatty acids. Many margarines contain these harmful fats, but manufacturers have not been required to list them on the label. (This practice is now being reviewed and they may be listed in the future.) The way to avoid them is to choose a margarine that states that there are no trans fats contained in it.

So how do you get the fats you need without feeling that you take your life in your hands every time you lift your fork? A good rule of thumb is to limit your fat consumption to thirty grams a day and to eat a minimum of twenty-five to thirty grams of fiber each day. With this diet, you can really eat until you're stuffed and it won't hurt you.

YOUR METABOLIC RATE

We've been referring throughout this chapter to your metabolism, the total amount of energy you use every day. There are three ways that you make use of this energy. Your basal metabolism burns up calories just keeping your basic systems, such as breathing and digestion, in operation. Basal metabolism is your energy rate while resting, the amount of energy, in calories, that you need to use up just to stay alive. It accounts for about 70 percent of the calories you use every day. Men burn from 1,400 to 1,900 calories a day in this process, while women burn between 1,000 and 1,500 calories. Size also matters: The larger and taller you are, the higher your basal metabolic rate.

You also use up energy in the process of digestion. And finally, you need energy to perform all your physical activities.

You know that if you take in more fuel—food—than you can burn up and convert into energy, you will gain weight, and that the reverse will take pounds off. But that's not the whole story. The *rate* at which you process that fuel and convert it to energy has a significant effect on your weight-control plan. *If you can increase your metabolic rate, even for short periods during the day, you will burn more fuel and store less of it in the form of fat.*

To a great extent, your metabolism is determined by your gender, your age, and even whether you are a night or morning person. But many people mistakenly believe that their basal metabolic rate cannot be altered. In fact, there's quite a bit you can do about it. Many research studies show you can favorably alter your metabolism to a maximum of about 10 percent, enough to allow you to burn several hundred extra calories a day.

Dieting, the centerpiece of the weight-control plan used by most Americans, induces your body to cannibalize muscle tissue for fuel rather than the stored fat that people hope and assume burns off because they've cut the amount of fuel coming in by cutting calories. When you drastically reduce your caloric intake, you're penalizing yourself because you are slowing your metabolic rate, discouraging further weight loss.

Dieting can lead to feeling deprived because you're not getting the food that you feel you want. But your body is also feeling deprived by the decrease in the number of total calories it has come to expect. It is actually shifting into starvation mode by slowing down your metabolic rate to hoard the calories you have already stored. Now you will burn up fewer of the calories coming in from your diet, and store a higher percentage of them as fat. That's why people often find dieting an increasingly frustrating way to slim down. The more you get into it, the more the dieting process itself makes it harder for you to lose weight.

What if you go on a calorie-reduction diet *and* increase physical activities? You may be able to hold off the phenomenon of muscle cannibalization to some extent because you are likely to be building new muscle. But your body is still going to feel deprived of its normal amount of fuel. You will have less energy for exercising at the same time you will need to work extra hard at staying physically active. Doesn't it make a lot more sense to both exercise and concentrate on eating the right foods, making sure that there's plenty of fiber in your meals so you won't be tempted to overeat, rather than simply cut calories?

Remember that what you eat also influences your calorie burn rate. If you want your metabolism to go full throttle, challenge it to work to the max. Eat foods that contain a moderate amount of protein and are lower in fat and higher in complex carbohydrates such as fiber-rich vegetables and whole grains. In other words, your most effective metabolic boosting diet is also the healthy one we advocate.

PLAY BALL ... PLAY ANYTHING

As we've mentioned, you can boost your metabolic rate by increasing muscle. The best way to accomplish this is to combine aerobic and resistance-type workouts, which improves cardiovascular health and helps control your weight.

Not only does exercise boost your metabolic rate while you're more physically active, but it also keeps the rate higher for hours afterward. That can mean burning an extra 25 to 200 calories a day (depending on the amount and kind of exercise you do) while you're doing nothing! If that doesn't sound like much, think of it as the more than 9,000 to 72,000 extra calories it would amount to over the course of a year. That's like getting a bonus of 2.5 to 20 pounds of weight loss every year over and above what you burn off while you're active. As they say, a few pounds here, a few pounds there, and before you know it. . . .

Increased physical activity, therefore, pays all kinds of dividends, improving your lung capacity, ensuring that your heart stays healthy, relaxing you, burning calories while you're active but also pushing your body to burn additional calories after you've finished with your activity.

The gist of it is that if you combine a good food plan with exercise, you're not only improving the fuel mix for your engine, but creating a better, more efficient engine as well. Significantly increasing exercise has a lot to do with that new you, and it is to exercise that we turn now.

CHAPTER 6

AEROBIC, STRENGTH, AND FLEXIBILITY EXERCISE

As we said at the beginning of this book, the best weight-control plan involves eating healthy foods (*not* dieting) and becoming physically active enough to at least offset the amount of calories you take in when you eat. That activity should range from the kind of aerobic and strength workouts that most people think of as "exercise," such as jogging and lifting weights, to low-level activities that are part of your everyday life, such as climbing stairs, to the calorie-burning movement called fidgeting that you can do at almost any time. Each has its place, emphasizing either intensity in small time slots or the ability to burn calories slowly but almost continuously throughout the day.

PUTTING EXERCISE IN ITS PLACE

The Mayo Clinic's Dr. Michael D. Jensen, the endocrinologist who was a principal author of the study that determined the newly discovered value of fidgeting in burning calories, put the place of exercise in weight control in perspective: "Exercise and diet are of equal importance, but if there's only one thing a patient can do, it's better they opt for exercise, because good exercise habits are usually maintained. Diets are not."

178

Unfortunately, most people have got it wrong, favoring dieting over physical activity. *The simple fact is that there is no better way to get rid of calories than to burn them off through increased physical activity.* Your level of physical activity is as much, or even more, likely to determine your weight pattern than what you eat. *The way to send that excess fat packing, instead of packing it in, is to get moving!*

That's good news. Overall it is likely to be easier for you to burn off the calories than to keep them from accumulating in the first place. Everyone has to eat. That puts you at the table several times a day, increasing the temptation to stray even if your willpower is pretty good. Exercise, on the other hand, as long as you are reasonably healthy, is completely within your control. You can do as much or as little as time and your inclination will allow. (Hopefully, you will want to do more than the minimum.)

But between schlepping the groceries, running errands, and taking care of the house and the kids, you probably get your fill of exercise, don't you? Not according to Dr. Donald D. Hensrud, a nutrition specialist at the Mayo Clinic. "Most people underestimate the number of calories they eat by about twenty percent—more if they're overweight," said Hensrud. "On the other hand, they overestimate their physical activity. It's not intentional or devious. It's just that we're not good judges."

The American Heart Association recommends that every adult, as a minimum, exercise for at least thirty minutes three or four times a week. In fact, at least six times a week for an hour daily is an even better recommendation.

Anyway you look at it, aerobic exercises—swimming, running, brisk walking—and weight and flexibility training are serious, heavy-duty weapons in your war on fat.

SEDENTARY NUMBERS

Despite a report from the surgeon general that exercise is a vital part of maintaining good health, Americans still do not give a high priority to physical activities.

- About 25 percent get *no* exercise.

- More than 60 percent get less exercise than the minimum recommended amount.

- The combination of poor diet and insufficient exercise ranks second behind tobacco as a cause of death in this country.

- If you don't exercise, your chances of getting cardiovascular disease increase by about 55 percent, your risk of developing high blood pressure rises 35 percent, and the chance that you will get a stroke may go up by as much as 50 percent.

First of all, they make for a stronger heart—no doubt, you know that. But they are also important because exercising can cause you to lose fat while you build muscle. Increasing your lean mass, the ratio of muscle to fat in your body, makes you more efficient when it comes to processing calories. It boosts your metabolic rate. The more muscle you have, the more calories you burn, even when you're sedentary, simply because muscle cells need to use more energy than do fat cells to sustain themselves.

One fear that many people have is that exercise makes you hungry, causing you to eat more and consume more calories than you would have if you had not bothered to exercise in the first place. You may be likelier to eat more because you exercise—although some people are less hungry because they work out—but it will not cause you to take in more calories than you burn off from the exercise. Exercise is calorie-efficient: You can't lose (anything except weight, of course).

Exercise is also your best friend when it comes to maintaining your weight, not just losing some. The people who have most success in sustaining initial weight loss are those who increase exercise in their daily-life routine.

What about the concept of your "set point" weight, an idea that has gained considerable attention in recent years? It holds that there is a natural weight level for you that, all things being equal, your body will try to return to if you take off pounds. Thus if you overindulge at the table, your body will work overtime trying to burn off the excess calories to get back to square one. More important for our purposes, it implies that if you take in fewer calories because you're eating a healthier diet, your body will lower its metabolic rate in an effort to push you back up to your starting point. Some studies do indicate the possibility of such a phenomenon. But even if it turns out to be true, additional exercise will counteract it, burning enough calories to maintain your new, lower weight.

TO YOUR HEALTH

You need exercise for some of the same reasons that your body requires protein in your diet. Exercise helps your body regenerate itself, repairing tissue when it wears down. It flexes tendons and joints, important at any age but even more so as you move into middle age, promotes a good night's sleep; helps ward off diabetes; and leaves you feeling more energetic. If you have diabetes, aerobic exercise will increase your sensitivity to insulin. If you have arthritis, exercise can improve your flexibility and hopefully reduce pain. Exercise also lowers your cholesterol—especially true of aerobic workouts—and may lengthen your life.

If you follow the health news in the newspapers, you know that we continue to discover new health benefits from exercising. The findings of one of the most recent reports, *The Nurses Health Study*, were that physical activity helps to prevent gallstones. If you've never had this condition and don't know someone who has, take our word for it: You don't want any part of it. From 10 to 15 percent of Americans eventually develop gallstones. Although they are often related to obesity, thin people can get them, too. But if you exercise regularly, you will substantially reduce your risk.

Besides cutting down your risk of developing cardiovascular disease, exercise is a factor in preventing osteoporosis because it strengthens your bones, promotes bone growth, and thus slows bone loss. Some studies also showed it reduces the risk of getting colon or breast cancer and that it lowers blood pressure. It can even improve your social life. Many people jog or work out in groups or in classes and end up making new friends and forming new romantic attachments.

Several recent studies at the University of Colorado confirmed the value of exercise in reducing and controlling stress. They bolstered earlier studies that indicated stronger immune defenses in people who exercised, and shorter illnesses when they did get sick. While the biological mechanisms relating exercise to stress reduction are still not totally clear, the end results are that if you exercise, you are simply likely to have a better day.

Exercise promotes mental health as well. By boosting the levels of important substances in your brain such as adrenaline, endorphins, serotonin, and dopamine, aerobic exercise helps fight depression. You're also likely to get a better night's sleep.

EXERCISE IS A WEIGHTY MATTER

The more you weigh, the more calories you will expend exercising for any given activity. So if you've allowed yourself to put on way too many pounds, as many of us do at one time or another, at least you can put them to work for you. Here's what you will burn in thirty minutes of swimming at a moderate pace using the crawl if you weigh

110 pounds	210 calories
123 pounds	234 calories
130 pounds	249 calories
143 pounds	273 calories
157 pounds	297 calories
170 pounds	336 calories
190 pounds	360 calories
223 pounds	423 calories

STAY AT IT AND ENJOY IT

What should you aim for in an exercise program? Before you even consider numerical goals, such as numbers of push-ups, bench presses, or miles run or walked, dedicate yourself to the idea that you are in it for the long run. The underlying spirit of what you are doing is consistency, to keep at it steadily. Your body will respond no better to an on-again-off-again exercise program than it will to the roller-coaster ride you give it by going off and on fad weight-loss diets.

In fact, we would go so far as to suggest that you think of being in it for good. Exercising at some level will work for you right into the latest of your later years. Recent research has been showing that the advantages of exercise seem to be there at any age. According to the National Institutes of Health, people in their nineties who worked out with weights were able to triple their leg strength and increase knee flexibility. There is reason to believe that regular exercise can give you a biological age equivalent to as many as twenty years less than your chronological age right up into old age. You will look it and feel it!

Your goal should be to incorporate physical activity into your life as a basic necessity, not as a luxury. You need to be physically active almost as much as you need to eat. But be realistic. If you've been leading a sedentary life, you are not going to build terrific muscle and lung power within the coming month. Start slowly, but, of course, it's okay to have ambitious goals in the back of your mind if there's a reasonable chance you will ultimately attain them.

Remember that you will be choosing activities that you will be doing an average of thirty minutes a day, some of them just about every day. They are going to become part of your life, so pick ones that appeal to you. This is not about suffering and sacrificing and being miserable because it's good for you. If that's what exercise turns out to be for you, you will eventually turn away from it. Find the right mix of athletics and pure exercise that fits your tastes and abilities and base your choice on whether facilities and equipment—if that's relevant—are readily available.

It's especially important that you don't get obsessed with what you are "supposed" to be doing. There is a whole range of physical activity that can bring you to your goal of losing and maintaining weight in a healthy manner. It doesn't have to be all push-ups and weight training—in fact, it doesn't really have to be any of that. Organizations such as the American Heart Association have confirmed that you can get the exercise you need by combining activities on the full spectrum of body movement, from the most traditional, to ones that don't even involve working up a sweat—we discuss them in detail in the next chapter—right down to the latest discovery, the everyday movement we have often dismissed as mere "fidgeting."

PLAY IT SAFE

If you have not been active, don't begin an exercise program without getting a physical checkup and discussing your plans with your doctor. There are many potential conditions, such as high blood pressure, that don't show themselves without medical tests and that might influence at least how you begin your program. If there are any doubts about your general health, check with your physician, and if you haven't seen one in a year, make an appointment just to be sure.

Always drink plenty of water every day, but especially before and after exercising. Your body requires about a cup of water for every 100 calories you burn. So if you've been jogging on a summer's day, it should take no feat of imagination to see why you need to drink up. If you've been drinking coffee or tea during the day, you will need to drink even more water, because caffeine, a diuretic, causes you to lose fluid.

It's a mistake to wait until you're thirsty to drink. Dehydration could already be under way by the time you crave a glass of water, so drink before, during, and after working out as a matter of course. Drinking water in the midst of exercise, by the way, should not cause cramps, no matter what you may have heard to the contrary.

CLOTHING

Except when you're taking your exercise lying down, as when you do bench presses, a good pair of exercise shoes

IF THE SHOE FITS . . .

Here's a tip to ensure a proper fit: The afternoon, when your feet have actually expanded a bit, is the best time to try on new shoes. Otherwise you could settle on a pair that's going to be a tad tight for a good part of the day.

will always be an asset. Try to wear the ones appropriate to the activity in which you're engaged and, of course, make sure they fit comfortably and provide adequate arch and heel support. Figure on needing new ones after running or walking 400 or so miles; at any rate, you will need a new pair before a year is out.

Common sense should dictate the kind of clothes you will wear: They should be comfortable and not fit too tightly. If you're going to exercise outdoors in cold weather, it's best to wear layers of clothing. Not only will they keep you warm enough, they will also permit you to shed layers once your metabolic rate picks up. Unless you have asthma, don't be afraid of the effect of the cold air on your lungs, by the way, unless it's cold enough to threaten you with frostbite (and then you wouldn't want to be out, anyway). The dry, cold air may feel a little harsh as you breathe it in, but your nose and throat will warm it before it gets to your lungs.

AEROBIC EXERCISE

Sometimes, with our understandable obsession with things that promote a healthy heart, it's easy to forget that the heart is first of all a muscle. It needs to be exercised beyond the times when it starts to pound because you spot an attractive stranger across a crowded room.

Your heart, like your other muscles, needs a regular workout. Aerobic activities such as walking, jogging, bike riding, and swimming, which force you to breathe harder, provide that exercise. Other things being equal—the absence of heart disease, for example—an older person's heart can work as well as that of someone half his age if he keeps it in good shape through aerobic workouts.

Aerobic exercise increases your blood level of HDL, the good cholesterol we discussed in the previous chapter. It also decreases your level of triglycerides, which are harmful fats, and enables your body to make more effective use of insulin.

While performing aerobic exercises, you will be burning up as much as twenty-five times the number of calories as you do at rest. Your heartbeat may nearly triple and the amount of air passing through your lungs can easily go from the 12 or so pints that course through them at rest to as many as 200. All in all, your body is doing quite a bit of work.

The fuel your body needs to provide this energy boost will initially come equally from stored fats and carbohydrates. After about twenty minutes or so, depending on how intensive your workout is, you will begin to burn more fats than carbohydrates. But don't get too caught up in this ratio. Your main aim should be to expend calories. Burn up more calories than you take in over a period of time and you will begin to make a substantial dent in that fat tissue. That's all that really counts for fat loss.

A question often asked about aerobic exercise is "Will I burn more calories walking or jogging slowly than if I move at a faster rate?" The answer is that it depends on how long you do it. For example, you can get the *same* caloric benefit from walking at four miles per hour for thirty minutes that you get from jogging at eight miles per hour for fifteen minutes. If you halve the intensity, you have to double the time; if you halve the time, you must double the intensity. We recommend covering more distance at a slower pace—this burns more fat calories.

All aerobic exercise involves a trade-off between the total time you work out and the intensity with which you do it. Stressing one or the other, time or intensity, is a matter of convenience, preference, and physical condition. For example, if your knees give you problems, walking, a lower-impact activity than jogging, is preferable. But you will have to spend more time walking than jogging to burn an equal number of calories to cover the same distance.

How do you know when you're working hard "enough" during a workout? The standard measurement of minimal aerobic activity is that you should be able to carry on a conversation even though you are breathing harder than when you are at rest. In a nutshell: You're exercising hard enough when you can talk but would find singing difficult.

To achieve substantial benefit from aerobic exercise, aim to do it at least thirty minutes per day, absolute minimum. Stay at it longer, for example, if you're walking at a moderate pace than you would if you were jogging. Some studies show that the benefits top out at a total of about 3½ hours per week.

TARGET HEART RATES

For good health, your aerobic workout should increase your heart rate, measured by your pulse. Check your pulse in any given exercise after doing it for about five minutes.

Take your pulse reading for about fifteen seconds after stopping, counting the beats. You can do this by placing three fingertips on your wrist on the thumb side. Move your fingertips around until you detect the throb of your pulse. Multiply the number of beats in fifteen seconds by 4 to get beats per minute.

The heart rate you should be shooting for is called your target heart rate, expressed in beats per minute. To find your target heart rate, subtract your age from 220. That gives you your maximum heart rate. Beginners should aim for a target rate range of 60 to 70 percent of this figure, moving up to 70 to 90 percent as they build endurance. Also be aware that these figures do not apply to swimming, because your heart slows down in the water, which means you must increase swiming intensity.

Remember, this is an approximate guide, not a principle etched in stone, and applies for cardiovascular health. For weight loss, the most important factor is total time of exercise.

WALKING AND JOGGING

Among all kinds of physical activity, 65 percent of Americans prefer walking. That's not surprising, since it is easy to do, requires no special equipment, is relatively low impact and thus adds comparatively little wear and tear to the body. Walking is cheap, and relatively easy to schedule, and the only equipment you need is a good pair of shoes. Shock-absorbing soles and insoles and a thumb's width between the end of the shoe and your big toe are important criteria in choosing a pair. You can walk for fitness and weight control even if you're on crutches or use a cane or even a walker. Walking is also a more effective way to burn calories than swimming or biking because you have to

EVEN IF YOU WALK, YOU'RE IN IT FOR THE LONG RUN

Walking and running are excellent ways of gradually reducing weight, but they won't do much in the short run. It will take thirty-five miles of either to work off the calories in one pound of body fat. But don't forget—the effects are cumulative. Just twenty minutes a day, and you'll begin to notice the weight loss sooner than you expect.

support your whole weight when you're on your feet. And because it's a weight-bearing exercise, walking helps to combat osteoporosis by helping to build bone mass.

The latest research suggests that ten-minute blocks of exercise work well. So if you can't find thirty minutes in a row to walk, do ten minutes at a time, as long as it adds up to three times during the day. Just ten minutes before and after dinner almost gets you to your minimum goal.

Even the slowest of walks, even strolls, can be helpful, especially after meals. Taking a long walk after dinner makes your metabolism more efficient. You can as much as double your metabolic rate, thus burning more of the calories from the food you've eaten before it can be stored as fat. While you don't have to walk fast, to derive this benefit you should begin within an hour of the end of the meal and keep going for at least twenty minutes. Such walks have an added advantage for those people who cannot seem to stick with a more formal schedule of longer walks for exercise. Walking twice a day after meals in effect breaks down their exercise into two shorter segments.

When walking for exercise, it's best to do it on flat, even ground, especially in the beginning, because steep hills can strain your muscles going down as well as up. If you want to walk on hilly terrain, get into it gradually. Your legs and feet will tell you when you are ready to pick up speed and increase the length of your exercise

RUNNING THOSE CALORIES INTO THE GROUND

The ultimate in burning calories by running would be participating in marathons. Such runners expend about 26 calories per minute for the duration of a race, which lasts more than two hours even for top-grade runners. Competitive athletes who train 100 miles a week for such races—and that's not unusual—burn 10,000 calories per week in the process. Olympic marathon runners who train year-round for four years burn more than 2 million calories, the equivalent of 555 pounds of body fat!

sessions. You can stretch before and after the walk, and warm up and cool down by strolling for a few minutes at the beginning and end of the session.

Swinging your arms a bit while walking increases the amount of physical activity you're getting during the walk and should provide you with a comfortable rhythm. Some people also like to hum while they walk. (There aren't any walking tunes that we know of, so hum what you like.) If you're ambitious, you can carry a small weight in each hand, increasing the benefits derived from this activity by upping the intensity of the exercise without increasing the pace. This is especially useful if your knees have been giving you any trouble, ruling out a fast-paced walk.

Another way of getting more out of walking is to do it through snow or on a beach. You will use up almost twice as many calories walking on wet sand as you would on a firm surface, and the resistance offered by hard snow is only slightly less. The view and the air quality are likely to be better, too.

SWIMMING

Among aerobic activities, swimming offers two significant advantages. First, the water supports your body, making it

CAN YOU GET A HEART ATTACK FROM JOGGING?

More than twenty years ago, author and runner Jim Fixx, who had done much to popularize jogging, died of a heart attack while running, raising this question for many people. One study followed almost 3,000 people who jogged and walked for exercise over a period of sixty-five months, covering approximately 375,000 hours of workouts. Two people had nonfatal cardiac problems, but nobody died. So the answer would seem to be that if you don't have a heart problem to begin with, the odds of aerobic exercise giving you one are extremely slim, while the odds of such workouts preventing heart disease are considerable. In fact, Jim Fixx had severe heart disease and did not know it. He probably lived as long as he did because he exercised.

a low-impact exercise that's very good for your back, knees, and feet if you are having problems in these areas. Second, you are also exercising almost all of your muscles simultaneously, and the resistance offered by the water and the need to use energy to maintain buoyancy means you are getting a high-calorie burn. In fact, over a given distance, you use up four times the amount of energy swimming as you do running.

As with any exercise, begin slowly unless you want to wake up the next day with terribly aching muscles and the prospect of staying high and dry for a week or two. Your eventual aim is to build up to a twenty-minute continuous swim. Vary your strokes throughout the swim, not only for variety but also to use as many muscles as possible. If you have any eye sensitivity to chlorine—assuming you're using a pool—wear goggles.

Remember that there's more to exercising in water than just swimming. Water aerobics have become enormously popular, especially for many people who have overdone such activities as aerobic dancing, or have done aerobics on surfaces that are too hard and have discovered what that can do to their knees and other joints. If this interests you, you can probably find a class at your club or gym or the local Y. Should you wish to work out alone, find a depth in the pool where the water comes no higher than midchest. This will provide you with all the support you need without affecting your ability to keep your balance.

AEROBIC DANCING

Aerobic dancing can be a lot of fun when done properly and it's something you can do with friends. Just make sure to do it on a soft enough surface. Decide beforehand that jumping will not be part of your workout and your knees will thank you. Here's a good rule of thumb: One foot should always be touching the floor.

If you are taking an aerobic dancing class, remember that the pace you keep has to be comfortable for you. If you feel you have some problem or weakness that might clash with what everyone else is doing, discuss it with the instructor so you can customize the routines for your body. Should you sense that the teacher is not too sympathetic to your needs, drop that class and sign up for another one.

STRENGTH TRAINING

Everyone should include at least some resistance training in their routine to build muscle. As we've pointed out, muscle tissue burns more calories to maintain itself, and when you lose weight, some of what's coming off will be muscle. Therefore you have to do something to at least replenish that muscle tissue.

WHAT'S THE MOST EFFICIENT WAY TO BURN CALORIES?

If you absolutely must have the very best in the way of intense exercise and you live in Miami, Atlanta, or Phoenix, you're out of luck. Minute for minute, cross-country skiing is the most intensive consumer of calories.

This becomes more important as you age. A woman at age sixty-five already has about twenty fewer pounds of muscle than she had when she was twenty-five. That adds up to 600 fewer calories burned per day simply because the proportion of fat to muscle tissue in her body has increased. All the more reason for older people not only to exercise but also to include strength training in their exercise programs.

People who don't exercise as they age will see their aerobic capacity halved between the ages of twenty and eighty. Metabolism also slows with age, by an average of 2 percent every ten years. If you allow your physical activity to slow down with it—according to the Mayo Clinic, 70 percent of older people are inactive—the decline in your metabolic rate could accelerate to as much as 5 percent per decade. No wonder that the average person gains about forty pounds, most of it fat, between the ages of thirty and seventy.

Studies have shown that men in the fifty to sixty-five age range can raise their metabolic rate at rest by about 8 percent by participating in strength training. The American Heart Association, the President's Council on Physical Fitness, and the American College of Sports Medicine are urging that people do some kind of strength training through all their adult years. There is no statute of limitations on "use it or lose it." (Although when it comes to muscle tissue and weight, perhaps we should really say "use it *and* lose it!")

Strength training, in addition to the obvious benefit of increasing your physical strength and giving you a more favorable ratio of muscle tissue to fat, will, like aerobic workouts, enhance your body's ability to use insulin to maintain an optimal level of glucose. It will also help you to lower your cholesterol, help check high blood pressure, strengthen your ligaments and tendons and enhance flexibility, and maintain bone mass.

Don't assume that you can do strength training only with barbells and dumbbells or costly machines. Many people get the same kind of benefit (working against resistance) from working with large latex bands that stress your muscles when you pull them. They're cheap, easy to store, and less likely to cause injury than heavier equipment. Handgrips are also inexpensive and help to diffuse tension as well as provide muscle-building exercise for your wrists and forearms. You can even make your own lightweight equipment by filling empty plastic beverage bottles with sand.

LIFT, PUSH, PULL, REPEAT

Strength exercises stress specific muscle groups. Ideally, you should aim to work on each group two to three times a week. Remember to warm up the muscle group you're exercising for about ten seconds before you begin the workout. Do a minimum of one set with eight to twelve repetitions of eight to ten different exercises at least twice a week. Performing one set develops as much strength as three sets! Breathe slowly, exhaling as you begin a repetition and inhaling as you complete it. Each rep should take about two or three seconds and be accomplished with as smooth a motion as possible.

Don't make the mistake that many people make of thinking that if a particular part of your body seems to have too much visible fat adhering to it, you can get rid of that fat by exercising the muscles near it. *There really is no spot fat reduction.* Exercising will reduce the size of fat cells throughout your body (the cells don't go away, they get smaller), and there is no way other than surgery that you can remove the fat from any one specific spot.

Exercising with good form is more than a matter of aesthetics. It can protect you from injury. In fact, it's more important to concentrate on good form than on the number of repetitions. Take your time, the time it takes to get it right.

FLEXIBILITY EXERCISES

While they don't get as much attention as aerobic and strength exercises, stretching workouts not only improve your body's flexibility, but may help to ward off injuries when you're doing those other kinds of exercises. Many calisthenics routines, such as half knee bends, bending to your right and left, and jumping jacks (on a mat or other soft surface, please!), constitute stretching. Try to fit such routines into your schedule three or more times a week and do them for a few minutes at a time.

Even if you are not among the millions (by some estimates, 80 percent of the adult population) who have at least some back pain, some of the most useful stretching exercises you can do are workouts aimed at strengthening the muscles that support the abdomen and back. They will help you to minimize debilitating back injuries.

Many of them are done lying down, always breathing easily and without holding your breath. Often they are meant to strengthen your abdomen, since those muscles are crucial for back support. Here are a few of the basic ones; hold each for five seconds:

- Lie on your back with your knees bent slightly and your feet flat on the floor. Pull your abdomen in and hold it in for five seconds. (Don't stop breathing!) Ten repeats should do it.

- In the same position, instead of just pulling in your abdomen, tilt it toward you as you pull it in. This is called the pelvic tilt. Repeat six to ten times.

- In the same position, place your hands on one of your knees and pull that leg back toward your chest slowly while tightening in your abdomenal muscles. Do six to ten repetitions first with one leg and then the other.

- Do another set of ten in the same manner, but this time pull both legs back simultaneously toward your chest. Remember, move slowly and don't arch your back or lift your head.

There is a whole aspect of stretching exercises that shades over into a world beyond workouts. Mind and body disciplines such as yoga and tai chi offer stretching routines and the benefits of psychological and even spiritual wellness. (We don't know anyone who couldn't use a little more stress reduction.) They can be customized to your needs and abilities. While classes are helpful, especially at the beginning, there are many good books that can guide you through doing it alone.

DO YOU NEED A GYM OR HEALTH CLUB?

There are advantages to working out at a gym or health club. Most of all, it's a structured environment in which everyone and everything around you, people and inanimate objects alike, are dedicated to working out. You can be inspired by those who are demonstrably working hard to get and stay in shape, and you will lack nothing you need in the way of equipment and advice.

What about trainers? True, they're expensive, and the gym or health club would very much like you to sign up for as many sessions as they can sell you. You're likely to be given at least one session on the house when you join. It could be a good idea to consider a few extra sessions to familiarize yourself with all the equipment and have the trainer work out a plan adapted to your needs so that you can make profitable use of the machines. Trainers can also help to get you motivated just when you may need a kick-start to incorporating exercise into the basics of your daily life.

Here's a tip if you feel a little lost the first time you are there *without* a trainer's supervision: Look around you. Almost certainly you will see other people doing what you had in mind for yourself. Watch them for a few minutes to see how they do it. Ask one of them questions if you're not sure of yourself (if he or she will just take off that Walkman long enough to hear you!).

Should you wish to work with a personal trainer outside of a gym or club, check his or her credentials. Two trustworthy organizations you can consult are the International Sports Science Association (ISSA), 1035 Santa Barbara Street, Suite 7, Santa Barbara, CA, 93101, (800) 892-4772, and the American College of Sports

Medicine (ACSM), P.O. Box 1440, Indianapolis, IN, 46206, (317) 637-9200.

If the gym or health club you joined or have considered joining does not look like a place at which you will be comfortable on a regular basis, remember many options are open to you. For example, there are Ys, community centers, colleges, and high schools that offer gym facilities, equipment, and exercise classes in the evening at reasonable rates.

HOME EXERCISE EQUIPMENT

Home exercise equipment certainly undercuts the "it's pouring (or snowing) outside and I don't feel like going to the gym" excuse for skipping an exercise session. But since these machines can range from a few hundred to a few thousand dollars each, it's a good idea to use them at the gym or at a friend's house before making a purchase.

The home exercise equipment industry is a $2 billion-a-year business. You will make a substantial contribution to this sum if you buy your own. So it behooves you to make sure you are getting what you want, need, and can use. Otherwise you could end up with a rather heavy, terribly oversized door stop or coat hanger.

If you buy a stationary bike, probably the most popular piece of home exercise equipment, consider one that offers the option of arm ergometers that will enable you to work the muscles in your upper body at the same time you pedal. You might also want to get one with electronic printouts that tells you how many calories you've burned so far, your distance traveled, and time spent exercising. If you need motivation, that should certainly supply it. Also remember when you're shopping: The heavier the bike, the better. Don't buy one less than sixty pounds.

Stationary bikes are especially useful when part of a larger aerobics routine. For example, you can use the bike to supplement walking or running, or let the bike be your principal means of aerobic work when the weather is terrible. Besides keeping it interesting, watching TV while "riding" is an easy way to both time your workout and schedule it. Just do it regularly when you watch a particular program.

If your bike has a gauge that measures revolutions per minute, begin with about 60 to 90. A good workout on a stationary bike lasts about half an hour, but don't hold yourself too closely to that. You don't want to negate the convenience of this equipment by making it into a chore. And remember that you can split up a session if the phone rings.

If you live in a walk-up, you probably don't need a stair stepper. Even the single flight of stairs in a two-story home should provide enough exercise of this type. Then again, you can't watch TV while actually going up and down the stairs. But if you can afford it, it's a great way to work out and burn extra calories.

Do you need a treadmill if you do a lot of walking outside? Well, it does offer the advantage of all-weather exercise, and we've never heard of anyone being chased by a dog when using one of these machines (unless they had neglected to feed their own pet). You also get to control the "terrain" you're walking on, something that's not going to happen on a road, street, or path.

Cross-country ski machines have an advantage over rowing machines: Skiing works the muscles in your upper as well as lower body, while rowing mainly stresses the upper. But be careful with both. Skiing machines, especially, really do give you a *work*out, maybe one that's more than you're bargaining for, and rowing machines can be

SIDEBAR: SWEATING IT OFF

According to the UCLA School of Medicine Obesity Clinic, the machines helping you to burn the most calories for any given amount of time using them are, in descending order, the treadmill, stair stepper, rowing machine, cross-country skiing machine, and stationary bicycle.

murder on a bad back and on your knees if your form is less than Olympic. Make sure that one of these is really for you before laying down the cash.

You need to be careful with free weights if that's your choice of equipment. They are, of course, heavy (why else would you want them?) and they can drop at the most inopportune times. Pay special attention to good form and observe all safety precautions. Before buying them, it's a good idea to work with a set under supervision of a personal trainer or at a gym or health club so you will be sure to know what you're doing. If you can afford it, you might want to consider buying a strength-training multiexercise machine as a safer alternative.

Working out at home is a little like working at home: You need to provide the kind of environment that will encourage you to stay focused. A good way to begin is to create a workout space near a mirror so that you can check your form, especially if you work with weights. Change into clothes that are suitable for what you are doing, just as you would if you were at a gym or health club. Motivate yourself by keeping a workout diary near your equipment to record your progress.

By all means, work out on a regular schedule. You will probably find it easier to keep at it if you know that you have a regular appointment to exercise. In fact, write it down on your calendar as if it were a meeting that can't be missed or rescheduled. Our rule of thumb: Unless the lottery calls to tell you you're a millionaire, don't let anything interfere with that appointment. No interruptions, not ever.

STAYING MOTIVATED

There are many things that might keep you from beginning an exercise program, but the most powerful is part of elementary physics: A body at rest tends to remain at rest unless acted upon by another force. If you've been enjoying life as a couch potato, bragging and making jokes about your aversion to sweat and exertion, and describing your idea of exercise as walking slowly to the nearest Burger King or Wendy's, you will need a force to overcome your inertia.

Chris Newton, a forty-six-year-old high school math teacher in Pittsburgh, was so set in his inert ways that his friends thought it would take the Force, à la *Star Wars,* to move him. In the end, what got him going was something considerably more powerful, the blood test results from his annual physical that showed a rise in his cholesterol to 320 from the 210 reading, near normal, recorded two years previously.

Fortunately most of us can get moving before life so dramatically intrudes. Some people are able to break down their resistance by putting it in writing, and if you are stuck before the starting line, you might want to try it. Write down all the feelings and obstacles that you think are holding you back. Then make a list of every reason you can think of why you want to get an exercise program for yourself going. Concentrate on what you would like exercising to do for you, and how you might feel if you achieved those goals.

But that's not the hardest part. The fact that you are reading this book says that you are already oriented to looking and feeling better, and that you understand increased physical activity must be part of the equation. It's *staying* motivated that's more important and harder than pushing yourself to begin. Since it's awfully easy to find excuses not to exercise for a few days—which inevitably stretch to more—whatever you can do to build motivation into your lifestyle and exercise program will work in your favor.

If you think that this is an exaggeration, consider your nearest gym or health club. If they've been doing their marketing, they've signed up hundreds of members. But the space and number of machines inside are limited. If everyone who plunked down $1,000 for a year's membership worked out as often as they intended to when they joined, most of their workouts would consist of standing in place, waiting on line to use the facilities.

GETTING STARTED

As with improving your eating habits, it's best to start when you are not under work or family pressure. That's why starting around the holidays is never a good idea. It's setting yourself up for failure. Certainly you want to begin when you're in good health. Once you start, ease into it. Otherwise you're setting yourself up for a muscle strain or worse and the beginnings of an ironclad excuse for dropping the whole thing.

Initiate your program with only a few repetitions if you're working with weights or on a machine at the gym. If it's aerobics, limit at first the distance you walk, jog, or swim and the time you spend doing it. Wait until it feels natural and routine before you start building up. This could take several weeks.

In fact, depending on your interests, you might start not with formal exercises but perhaps with a friendly, low-keyed game of handball, volleyball, or squash two or three times a week. Or you might edge into a walking routine by going window-shopping on your lunch hour, adding a few extra blocks in which you quicken the pace somewhat. This is especially important if you have really been sedentary. Just engaging in one kind of physical activity should make it easier to add others.

Working out or playing sports with friends is an excellent way to get yourself to "do it." There's nothing like having positive reinforcement and sharing the downs as well as the ups of any activity to get you to keep at it. If your activity is something you can do at a moderate pace, such as walking, doing it with someone else, talking all the while, will make the time fly by, make it more enjoyable, and create a social occasion to which you will look forward.

In addition to the companionship, you will be lending each other support and encouragement when motivation sags, as it will on some days for everyone. A bonus from making it a social activity is that if you're having a problem, say, with form, your buddy can watch what you're doing and help you to correct it.

Speaking of other people, a good way to motivate yourself, especially when you're first edging into exercising, is to pick out people you know who have the kind of persistence and long-term commitment that you would like to develop. Make role models out of these people— but don't feel that you *have* to match their repetitions or intensity or total time spent exercising. Ask what keeps them going and make it clear that you admire their stick-to-itiveness. There's a good chance that they will then take an interest in your success and be in your corner with support and help if you start to falter.

It wouldn't hurt, either, to read the weight-loss/exercise success stories in the Sunday supplements to your newspaper and in fitness magazines. Just keep in mind that some of these tales are a little stretched, and you don't have to be a superman or -woman and turn your life around on a dime to be a success.

If you're exercising alone, it's a good time to mull over some problem that has you stymied, such as whether or not to refinance your mortgage. Working out puts you into a kind of rhythm that is actually very conducive to problem solving and creative thought. By taking advantage of this phenomenon, you will make your exercise time more useful, productive, and valuable, one more reason to persist in doing it.

Another good motivator is an outfit you *hope* to fit into. Maybe that's a bathing suit, jeans, a new dress or pair of pants, or a form-fitting shirt. Hang it up in front of you as you work out at home or take a mental picture so you can envision yourself in it as you sweat off the calories at the gym.

One way you can remind yourself of why you're pushing yourself to do something strenuous, even on a "bad" day, is to keep an old piece of clothing around that dates from your thinner days. Place with it a pair of pants from your current size as you begin to lose inches, to show yourself that you've made progress.

Did you ever keep a diary? Try one devoted solely to exercising. Jot down how it went that day and how you felt about yourself as a result of the workout. Remember

A FRIENDLY GAME OF . . .

The quintessential way to burn calories and have fun is to play a sport with friends. Here's what just a half hour of playing these sports will be worth to you if you weigh 150 pounds:

Basketball: 286 calories
Bowling: 107
Touch football: 286
Golf: 161
Racquetball: 358
Skiing: 250
Soccer: 250
Tennis: 250
Volleyball: 107

to frequently remind yourself, in writing, of why you need to keep at it. Every once in a while look back at your entries. It can help you to spot negative patterns of thought and perhaps notice any apparent connections between feeling resistance to exercising and what was going on in your life that day.

You might also try the mirror image of the exercise diary: the sedentary log. Simply keep track of all the time you spend sitting during the week. That might motivate you to get going.

If you're exercising outside—jogging or walking, for example—keep a sheltered activity in reserve for a rainy day (see the next chapter for ideas). That's one of the best ways to avoid the danger of the "act of God" excuse.

VARIETY

Even if you hit a string of sunny, mild days, vary your routine so you don't get bored. If you're lifting weights, add enough exercises to your repertoire so that you're rarely do the same sets of the same things two weeks in a row. If it's running or walking, take a different route. By the way, did you ever notice how different a street can look if you walk up it rather than down? If you travel the same route but begin from the other end, whether walking for exercise or jogging, you will be on a seemingly different street. Just try it.

Along the same lines, don't exercise at precisely the same time every day. If you usually jog after work, for instance, maybe do some chores around the house and walk the dog before you run, not after. That little bit of variety will put a different cast on the day.

If you find that your routines are becoming too routine, write down all the possible ways you could get your exercise in during the week without repeating yourself. This is what the American Heart Association calls a "fitness menu," a list that can range from walking and biking to rowing and lifting weights. There are almost certainly more things to do than you realize, and writing them down will bring them front and center.

KEEP ON TRACK

Everyone hits a slump once in a while. That could manifest itself as taking off too many days from your exercise program. If that happens, here's a way to reorient yourself toward your goal. Aim to have one "perfect" day of nutrition and exercise where you bear down and do everything right. Choose the day so that it's not one where you have a deadline or have to deal with a pressing personal problem—you want a formula for success, not failure. You don't have to keep up that pace of perfection every day, but slipping in a day like that when you've begun to slack off, and then maybe increasing it to two or more days in a row, is a great way to remind yourself that doing the right thing is not that hard, and that if you can do it one day, you can do it most, or at least many, days as well.

Ultimately, time is on your side. The longer you exercise regularly, the more it becomes an integral part of your life. Before you know it, it will seem the "natural" thing to do. For most people, that happens after about six weeks. Then if you get sick and miss a few days, you really will *miss* them. When you reach that point, you've just about got it made.

WHEN DAILY LIFE GETS IN THE WAY

Aerobic, strength, and flexibility training are the bedrock of physical fitness and the big guns in the war on weight when it comes to physical activity. For a fortunate few who have the time and the dedication, these activities, combined with a healthy diet, are enough to do the job. But for most of us, they provide the foundation on which we need to add something else.

We need something else for no other reason than life has a funny way of intervening to keep us short of our goals for exercising. Your report is due on Monday. There go two days of jogging. Your spouse's car is on the blink, in the repair shop, and unavailable. You won't make it to the health club anytime this week. The organized volleyball game you've relied on this fall is off for two weeks because someone's sick and a few people are going to be out of town.

But you are certainly not going to stop eating in the meanwhile. How will you keep burning off those calories? Until recently, most weight and fitness plans skirted this issue. Not anymore, as you will see in the next chapter.

CHAPTER 7
NO SWEAT: MOVE MORE, MOVE OFTEN, JUST MOVE!

PHYSICAL ACTIVITIES THAT MAKE YOU SWEAT AND substantially quicken your breathing are *invaluable* to your health. We hope we've convinced you of this basic truth. Over time they will make you look better, too, burning calories and helping you to shed pounds—especially when accompanied by eating healthier foods. We strongly recommend that to the extent possible—given the demands on your time and your general health—that you try to engage in a program of aerobic workouts and weight training, with machines or free weights.

But let's also be real. We don't live in an ideal world, and for many people, our modern lifestyle simply works against what one "should" be doing. A recent study at Harvard made this dramatically clear. On the one hand, research based on the lifestyles and health habits of more than 84,000 middle-aged female nurses showed that the chances of getting heart disease decreased by a stunning 82 percent if a person followed all the health guidelines published in recent years involving not smoking, eating the right diet, and getting enough exercise. The bad news is that among this group of nurses, who should have been more aware of these guidelines than most people, only 1 percent fully complied with the well-known prescriptions for good health.

But if ever we needed to pay more attention to fitness and health, it's now. In October 1999, the U.S. Centers for Disease Control and Prevention released a study, published in *The Journal of the American Medical Association*, that had some disturbing implications for those who had hoped that the healthy diet and exercise message might be getting through to the public. The study, based on a sample of 100,000 participants chosen at random, reported that between 1991 and 1998, obesity (more than 30 percent above ideal body weight) had increased by almost 18 percent in the American population. The largest weight gain was found among people in their twenties.

The authors of the report noted that the amount of physical activity that people were getting had not increased at all in that time, with the implication that people are probably getting more careless with their diet without compensating with more exercise. "Rarely do chronic conditions such as obesity spread with the speed and dispersion characteristic of a communicable disease epidemic," the authors concluded, with alarm.

THE WAY THINGS USED TO BE

With modern technology and our tendency to adopt passive entertainment, most of us don't take advantage of the chances literally surrounding us to conveniently burn calories. It wasn't always like that. At one time, you didn't need a gym or exercise equipment, all you needed was daily life and its physical requirements.

In the past 125 years, the amount of work it has taken just to get through the day has decreased more than it did in the previous 3,000 years. They didn't need to do moderate exercise in post–Civil War America because it was embodied in daily life. Chopping, hauling, lifting, and pushing characterized the day.

In truth, even then some new technology was penetrating the kitchen. For example, housewives had access to coffee grinders and eggbeaters—but they were worked by hand. The same held for the first washing machines, which had to be laboriously, almost painfully cranked. But most people did laundry the way it had been done for several thousand years—at a nearby stream or with water hauled from there or from a well to the house. Needless to say, once washed, clothes had to be hung out to dry and then gathered from the line.

Although the cooking stove had replaced the open hearth in the middle of the room, it was still likely to be fueled by wood, which had to be chopped, or coal, which the homeowner had to carry from the coal bin. The pots on the stove were big and heavy and were used to heat water for both cooking and bathing. Some houses had pipes to carry that water to sinks and tubs for dish washing and bathing, but most people still had to carry the hot water to the tub, pail by pail.

If you lived in the country, you might have access to fresh fruits and vegetables in season from your own garden. But that meant they were cultivated, picked, and cleaned by hand, although commercially canned food was beginning to become available. Urban dwellers could buy the raw food for meals in stores, with the emphasis on the "s." For the great majority of people, one-stop shopping in supermarkets was still unknown—the first A&P supermarket opened in 1864 and fifteen years later there were still only about 100 in the whole country. Virtually everything was made from scratch and during the warmer months, there was the extra job of canning produce so that it would be available in some form come winter.

With streets dirtier than they are today, tracked-in dirt was a major problem. The solution was broom power, supplied by one's upper arms. Carpet sweepers were just making their appearance, but they were still a luxury. If it was time to clean the rug, you dragged it outside, draped it over a clothesline, and beat the dickens out of it.

So who needed a gym or personal trainer? Your "abs" could stay hard as a rock and your waistline be permanently held in check—*if* you just laid off the lard, pies, and biscuits on the dinner table and managed not to raise eight or nine children.

WHERE WE'RE AT

Clearly we are in a different place. Modern life often conspires to keep us from getting enough vigorous exercise. A lack of time is a major factor. Other reasons are plain tiredness and the distractions of home entertainment after a day's work. How can you get that physical activity you know you need, given your lifestyle? What can you do to burn enough total calories to offset the ones that come in at mealtime?

Aside from the times we live in, there's always the problem that from the perspective of diet and exercise, we're only human. Had a bad week? Did you drop out for a while from the battle of the waistline? It's so discouragingly easy to backslide, and such backsliding has a way of building itself permanently into your life. *If you so much as burn 100 calories per day less than you had been consuming but continue to eat the same diet, you would put on ten pounds in*

CAN YOU THINK YOURSELF THIN?

As you might have suspected, thinking does use energy. Unfortunately, the amount is minuscule and you would end up with quite a headache before you had anything corporeal to show for it.

one year. That's all it takes—a little slackening off that you might hardly notice.

If you also build that kind of slight drop-off in activity into your lifestyle, it can produce that dreaded middle-age spread almost by itself. Even if you had been only mildly active and then became sedentary, it could easily result in your expending 100 fewer calories per day. Add that to the 100 calories per day extra you've been adding at the dinner table and suddenly you are looking at a weight gain of twenty pounds per year. Add on a couple of years, and the mirror and your waistline will be giving you some very bad news.

GOOD NEWS!

That's enough doom and gloom. Here's what you need to know about recent studies showing that lifestyle adaptations—increasing physical activity short of sweaty workouts—can help you to keep your weight under control and improve your health.

One study, conducted by Dr. Stephen Blair at the Cooper Institute for Aerobics Research in Dallas and published in *The Journal of the American Medical Association*, involved more than 200 slightly pudgy individuals of both sexes, ages thirty-five to sixty, who engaged in virtually no exercise. They were placed into one of two groups. Half were sent into the gym for thirty minutes of aerobics five days a week, while the others were assigned to integrate activities such as stair climbing and moderate walking into their daily routines, forgoing elevators and their cars. After two years, both groups had better cardiovascular fitness than when they started and both groups had shed body fat (but *not* weight—they didn't change their diets). The eye-opening fact is that the lifestyle adjustments produced results on a par with structured exercise. Members of each group had worked off body fat while building better musculature. Imagine if they had combined these activities with a better diet!

Given our sometime obsession with hard exercise—formally structured workouts that leave you sweaty—these findings are potentially revolutionary. But only if people are willing to keep to a regular schedule of thirty minutes a day of moderate exercise in place of, or better yet, in addition to the heavy stuff. Or as Dr. Ross Anderson, who led a similar study at Johns Hopkins, said in a January 1999 Associated Press article of these new revelations about the value of moderate exercise, it can't be done too casually, "with ten minutes on Monday and ten minutes on Tuesday." Even moderate exercise, Anderson cautioned, "has to be done at a purposeful pace."

The study at the Johns Hopkins University School of Medicine involved women who were substantially overweight. In this case, the participants were given a diet as well as assignments to either aerobic workouts or lifestyle modification. They maintained these programs for sixteen weeks. The results were similar reductions in weight for both groups. But here's the significant part: *After one year, it was the walkers and stair climbers, not the joggers, who had put back the least amount of weight.*

The team conducting the research concluded: *"Patients should strive to incorporate regular physical activity into their lives on a daily basis but should realize that even some physical activity, even if not performed regularly, is much better than being sedentary."* In fact, people are more likely to stay with "exercise" that is not seen as exercise. They *are* more likely to do it regularly.

Dr. Michael Pratt of the Centers for Disease Control put the message in even more immediate and personal terms. *"People have choices,"* he pointed out in a July 1999 *New Choices* article, "that's the most compelling message that comes out of these studies."

These findings empower all of us. They give the kind of low-level exercise embodied in our daily activities an even greater importance. People who are alert to the calorie-burning opportunities that are within arm's (and leg's) reach during the day have a chance to insert exercise periods into their lives where time slots for such activity don't even appear to exist. They have a good chance to do at least the minimum daily exercise recommended by groups such as the American College of Sports Medicine and the American Heart Association, and perhaps more. And they can do it without disrupting their lives. In fact, even people who faithfully set aside and use formal exercise time every day can benefit from lower-level exercise.

As studies such as these have revealed the fitness value of any physical activity, the Centers for Disease Control, the American College of Sports Medicine, and the American Heart Association have incorporated their findings into what they recommend as a minimum of activity to maintain health and fitness. This activity stresses duration and frequency over intensity. Currently they advise everyone to spend at least *thirty minutes a day, every day*, in moderate activity—brisk walking, for example, or bicycling, or even washing the car or dancing. *Just move at*

ANOTHER PYRAMID

Graduate students in the Department of Kinesiology and Health at Georgia State University have taken the new importance given to low-level exercise and have illustrated it with a pyramid comparable to the Department of Agriculture's food pyramid. At the bottom, making up the foundation, are the low-level, everyday activities we've discussed in this chapter, such as washing and waxing the car, walking the dog, walking to do your errands, and mowing the lawn. Above them is high-intensity exercise—aerobic, strength, and flexibility—that you really need but don't have to spend quite so much time doing. Above it, useful two to three days per week, are games and activities such as hiking, bowling, golf, and yoga. On top, marked "Do sparingly" (like the pies, pastries, and ice cream at the tip of the food pyramid) are computer games, every labor-saving device you can think of, and, of course, the ubiquitous TV.

We don't necessarily hold to every detail in their diagram. For example, you can profit from and enjoy athletic activities just about every day. And these students devised their pyramid before the new information about the power of fidgeting became available. But by and large they are on the right track, and you will be, too, if you generally stick with their scheme.

a decent pace. Even if your day is heavily scheduled, there's hardly an excuse for not doing this because *the thirty minutes can be broken up into as little as ten-minute segments.* Just make sure that those segments eventually add up to thirty minutes or more every day.

You may not believe it right now if you've been inactive, *but you have it in you to do what you need to do to get into better shape and better health without bending your life out of shape.* According to Dr. Martin Katahn, former director of the Weight Management Program at Vanderbilt University, "There lies sleeping in the most sedentary body a capacity for moving around, bending, flexing, and playing that, once developed and expressed, satisfies some basic biological need and gives unparalleled pleasure."

THE STARTING POINT

Even if you've been sedentary, you're not starting from absolute zero. You're never doing "nothing," although you might think you are. Even sitting quietly burns calories—about 1.5 per minute, or 90 or so an hour if you weigh about 150 pounds (although that's still less than the number of calories you would take in from eating something so innocuous as a rice cake). Just standing around, you expend 1.8 calories a minute. Even when you're showering and dressing in the morning, you are burning an average of about 3.3 calories a minute.

Nevertheless, at that rate you're not likely to get too far ahead of the incoming calories from even a bread-and-water diet. But now let's pick up the pace. Look at the calorie-burning benefits you get from these common activities, according to the UCLA School of Medicine Obesity Center. The first number is calories per minute, the second, calories burned per hour, and the numbers are for a person who weighs about 150 pounds:

Activity	Calories burned per minute	Calories burned per hour
Window shopping	3	180
Ballroom dancing	3.5	210
Gardening	4	240

(continues)

Activity	Calories burned per minute	Calories burned per hour
Carpentry	4	240
Washing the floors	4.2	252
Golf (no cart)	4.3	260
Tennis	6.6	386
Swimming	8.5	510
Moderate aerobic workout	9.2	552
Climbing stairs	11	660

Two things are significant about these numbers. The first, not surprisingly, is that the more intense activities certainly burn more calories in any given time. But the second suggests the calorie-burning possibilities inherent in such activities as dancing and housework if you did enough of them and their like throughout the day. There are workouts and there are workouts. We hope to convince you that you can virtually build day-long "routines" using low-level exercise to supplement and, if necessary, replace formal exercise. The key, again, is to *keep moving.*

AROUND THE HOUSE

Sandy Alderston couldn't figure it out. A housewife with a two-year-old daughter living in Greenville, North Carolina, Sandy thought she had a pretty busy day, between taking care of her child, shopping, cooking, and cleaning. Yet although she watched her diet and even went to the gym several times a week when she could get a baby-sitter, she couldn't quite keep her weight in check. It would drift up to seven or eight pounds over the level it had been for years, and she had a devil of a time getting back down to a manageable number. She only accomplished that by temporarily depriving herself at dinner of some of the dishes she liked most, like pasta.

There are a lot of people like Sandy who just miss gaining control of the way they look. They really could use something beyond working out and riding herd on themselves at the table. Does that ever sound like you?

Often, without realizing it, we have calorie-burning resources we pass up, even in the midst of what we think is an active life. The trick is just to become more aware of how you interact with your physical environment.

The day is long, and so are your muscles: Use both to your advantage. For instance, watching TV doesn't have to mean total physical downtime. You could be straightening up the living room or dusting while the box is on. By the same token, you could be folding the wash upstairs instead of on the ground floor. The clothes won't look any cleaner for the extra height, but you will burn at least 25 calories carrying them up the stairs.

While doing the wash, you could work some informal, ad hoc calisthenics into the chore. For example, in taking the clothes from the washing machine to transfer them to the dryer, squat, bending your knees, as you shovel them into the dryer, then stand up to your full height, walk over to the washing machine, grab another bunch, and repeat.

However often you do such chores as vacuuming, you might consider doing them more often for their calorie-burning benefits. In fact, the movements you use to clean with a vacuum cleaner are quite close to those you would employ with a rowing machine. The difference is that the rowing machine offers considerably more resistance and thus enhances your ability to burn calories in a shorter amount of time. But you could compensate for the intensity with increased time with the vacuum cleaner. It's also possible to increase your consumption of calories while vacuuming by adding complexity to the task. For instance, put some music on the stereo and then move as if you were dancing with the appliance. It's okay, no one is watching.

If you care for a young child, you don't need us to tell you how many calories that can burn! But you can enhance the number of calories you burn and literally get closer to your child if you use a backpack or frontpack to carry the child around instead of a stroller. A 130-pound woman making use of this basic form of transportation will burn about 350 calories in an hour, about twice as many as she would pushing a stroller and as many as she would consume playing doubles tennis.

Have you been paying one of the kids on the block to rake your leaves or mow your lawn? We're not suggesting that you put a child who wants to earn spending money out of work. But you could be raking alongside, burning calories as you go, and it could be you behind that lawn mower, and the boy or girl from across the street could be doing something else for you while you're at it.

The same goes for cleaning the house if you hire someone to do it every week or so. Find some projects that you've been putting off and work alongside the cleaning person to get more done than would otherwise be the case. You will burn calories and have a feeling of accomplishment, too.

Your garden, of course, is a veritable gym supplied by nature if you will take advantage of it. A half hour devoted

GETTING MOWED DOWN

Using a manual lawn mower rather than a motorized one not only is beneficial from the point of view of fitness, but also makes America a safer place. As many as 400,000 people a year are injured by the noisier variety of mowers, with the eyes at greatest risk. That's not surprising, since objects caught in the mower's blades can be propelled outward at speeds of 200 miles per hour. In 1997, mower-caused injuries were serious enough to bring 60,000 people to hospital emergency rooms.

By the way, we, of course, mean a lawn mower without a seat to make it a sedentary activity. In fact, if you're up to it, a manual lawn mower is the best for getting a workout while you trim the grass. If you have a very big lawn, perhaps use a power mower to get most of it, but always save a patch you can cover with an old manual model.

The nonmotorized lawn mower offers an advantage in addition to helping you burn more calories: It's quiet. If you are one of those people who like to take care of chores early in the day, you will be positively empowered by a manual model, which won't disturb the neighbors.

Do you need some numbers to be convinced? Here is what you can burn in 30 minutes of lawn mowing:

Seated: 101 calories

Pushing a motorized model: 182 calories

Pushing a manual mower: 243 calories

to planting seeds, for instance, burns about 160 calories. Weeding uses up 182 and planting seedlings consumes about 160. If you feel ambitious (and need to fill a fireplace), there's always chopping wood, which will burn off about 250 calories in thirty minutes.

You have to wash your car, don't you? Why pay to have it done when doing it yourself provides a good, vigorous workout involving stretching, squatting, and bending—great flexibility enhancers—and can become a good family social occasion if shared between spouses and children?

Even if you think you're doing just about as much as you possibly could at home in the way of staying active, "it ain't necessarily so." Alan Shugart thought he was positively a whirlwind around the house. He crammed the weekends with do-it-yourself project work in the garage to the extent that his wife thought she would have to take up auto repair and maintenance just to spend time in the same room with him. The problem was that most weekends last only two days and Alan was constantly falling short of his goals, finding himself with incomplete projects, some of which he never finished because during the week, he lost the impetus that usually seized him on Friday evenings.

Alan's problem was that he was becoming fixated on Saturdays and Sundays. Finally he found a solution that you might be able to adapt to whatever interests you. He simply began to apportion a share of the work to weekday evenings. He scheduled it so that he did a little bit just about every day. By doing this, he kept up the momentum that he built on weekends, actually finished more of the projects, and burned a significant number of calories while he was doing something that he now enjoyed even more than before.

"YOU SHOULD BE DANCING"

The musical group the Bee Gees had some good low-level exercise advice on the soundtrack of the film *Saturday Night Fever:* "You Should Be Dancing." You don't even need a partner. Anytime you find yourself with ten minutes to spare, just slip a CD onto your stereo and let it all hang loose. A 145-pound woman can burn 50 calories enjoying this kind of break in the day. The soundtrack we just mentioned from *Saturday Night Fever* is excellent for this purpose—hear it and just *try* to stay still! The soundtrack from *Flash Dance* (especially "What a Feeling!") is another good bet, as is the score from the film *Fame*. Of course, there's always Motown, with that oh-so-danceable beat. But follow your own tastes—disco, rap, whatever—just get up off the couch and boogie away those calories.

For couples, dancing is great for exercise, not to mention what it can do for the relationship. "It's the ultimate togetherness workout," as Phil Martin, a dance instructor at California State University at Long Beach put it. "You move in a physical harmony that works toward an emotional harmony." And when the dancing is vigorous, as in swing dancing or salsa, there's a definite aerobic benefit from the elevation of your heart rate. A study at the University of West Australia that concentrated on the rumba discovered that the Cuban dance could offer an aerobic workout comparable to running.

If you own your own home, or rent or own an apartment on the ground floor, you are likely to have gardening opportunities that you don't fully utilize. That ground outside is just dirt if you don't cultivate it. Grass is fine, but there's always room for some variety, color, and maybe even a vegetable or two that would look great on a salad plate. Survey what you've got. Bet you can see possibilities for plantings. Once you take advantage of the opportunities, you will have a rewarding exercise that will work many muscles for much of the year, and one of the greatest kinds of satisfaction that physical activity can ever deliver.

THE ROOTS OF CARDIAC HEALTH

A study at the University of Washington Cardiovascular Health Research Unit showed that at least an hour of gardening a week reduced the chances of getting a heart attack by 66 percent when compared with people who did not exercise.

A word of caution, though: Stretch before you dig. You could injure your back if you plunge into gardening without properly limbering up.

Are family values important to you? What could be more family oriented than playing with your children in the backyard or in a nearby park (to which you may also be able to walk and burn calories even before you get there). Even just "horsing around" with the kids outside provides good fitness benefits for you and your children. However, any formally structured game you could think of might be even better, since it's likely to extend the time you will be active and perhaps make it even more fun. It doesn't have to be anything fancy or complicated. For example, a 135-pound woman will expend almost 100 calories just playing Frisbee for thirty minutes, while a 175-pound man will use up 125 in the same amount of time. A woman at that weight will burn a little over 160 calories in something more strenuous, such as tag, while the man will consume upward of 200.

You could get some good exercise in and score a lot of points with your children if you volunteer to improve their playtime. If they're learning to play tennis, for example, you could be the one who fetches stray shots that go off the court. Is baseball their sport? Hit fly balls to them or catch them if they want to hit. Maybe they need a temporary goalie so they can practice for soccer. You could also stand under the basket while they shoot hoops, chasing down the rebounds and passing the ball back to them so they can shoot again.

There are so many ways you can play with the kids and benefit from all the physical activity yourself. For example, when was the last time you tried skipping? Probably not since elementary school. Skip around for about fifteen minutes and if you weigh 150 pounds, you're knocking off about 85 calories—and your kids will be talking about it to their friends for a week or two afterward.

Don't leave the dog out of the fun, by the way. Adding a four-legged creature to the mix will always create more movement, although it's impossible to say in advance who might end up chasing whom.

OUTDOORS AND AWAY FROM HOME

How often have you driven yourself to distraction trying to find a parking space reasonably close to the stores at the mall? Why? Here's a perfect opportunity to squeeze a walk into your day where there wasn't time for one before. You could view the scarcity of prime parking spaces as an opportunity rather than as an obstacle. Yes, there are more scenic places to walk, but you could put this stroll to good use, aside from its calorie-burning and muscle-toning potential. Use the time it takes to get to the door to think about what you want to buy and what you need to resist picking up on impulse. Clear your head in this way and you are less likely to discover afterward that you had unintentionally cleared your wallet.

Dr. Miriam E. Nelson, director of the Tufts University Center for Physical Fitness, formulated a good general rule about when to use the car. She suggested that every time you reach for your car keys, you should ask yourself, "Can I do this using my own muscles and energy without getting in the car?" Perhaps you can drop something off at a friend's house using a bike. Do you really need four wheels to mail that letter? Even if you are taking your son or daughter somewhere, might it be close enough for you and your child to walk there and back together? You could be getting him or her into some good habits as well as burning calories yourself. It could also be a great opportunity to have a leisurely conversation with that very important young person.

Even when you feel you don't have so much time to spare for walking, it could turn out to be a more efficient way of getting around than you had thought. You should be able to walk two miles in thirty minutes when going full tilt. If you were in a car and got caught in traffic, you might not do much better than that, and then you might still have to spend some time finding parking.

Malls themselves also provide exercise opportunities beyond just walking from store to store and within stores. Surely you've noticed people purposefully walking through the mall without pulling out a credit card. Mall walking, with or without others in a group, is a good way to get in your daily thirty minutes of physical activity, or at least a substantial part of it. It's especially useful in areas so heavily built up and given over to the auto that finding good and safe places to walk is a problem. Mall walking is also a good alternative to walking outside in inclement weather. Keep that in mind even if purposeful walking in the mall rather than just shopping is not part of your usual physical activity routine.

Most supermarkets offer the option of pushing a cart or grabbing a basket. If you're not shopping for the whole

TWO LEGS VS. TWO WHEELS

Even a leisurely walk can give you a better calorie burn than you might expect. Walking three miles per hour will consume almost as many calories as biking the same distance at six miles per hour— about 186 calories for a 110-pound individual.

week, always choose the hand-held basket. As with mall shopping, there's the added benefit of being less inclined to buy things on impulse because you will actually feel everything you put in the basket, encouraging you to ask yourself if you really need and want it.

Once you're finished grocery shopping, you could push your purchases back to your car in a cart. But even if you get one where the wheels don't lock and make you frustrated, you're missing a great chance for a mini-workout. Just pick up the packages and go! Most likely they won't weigh *that* much, but if they do, you could at least have some in the cart while you carry the others in one hand, switching off hands every fifty feet. You would be amazed at how much you could work off even with that over the course of several months.

If you're like most Americans, you've become thoroughly comfortable with shopping for groceries in megamarkets with acres of parking space. But that's not the only way you can buy your food. There are plenty of convenience stores in every part of the country. If you live in a city, there are probably small food stores you can reach without ever going near a highway. Whenever possible, walk to one of these stores for staples like milk and bread. Yes, the prices may be a bit higher than in the supermarket, but you will probably buy only a fraction of your groceries there and the fitness benefits will far outweigh the

BIT BY BIT

Walking off calories can be divided into really small segments. Dr. Tom Birk, who teaches physical medicine, rehabilitation, and physical therapy at Wayne State University, points out that even a three-minute walk at three miles per hour disposes of 10 calories for a 130-pound woman. Now imagine doing that many times a day just about every day. If you live in a two-story home, don't pass up the opportunity to walk upstairs at the slightest excuse. That same 130-pound woman could knock off 17 calories each time she climbs that one flight.

few pennies more you spend. You are also more likely to be able to chat with the people behind the counter than you would in those football-field-sized stores.

UP AND DOWN, BACK AND FORTH

Do you encounter escalators during your day—at work or shopping? How about using them to escalate the number of calories you burn, rather than just standing there while the world moves by? Of course, you can walk up the stairs instead. But almost always, assuming the escalator is wide enough, people will move over to the right to permit others in a hurry (or those interested in being more physically active) to pass them on the left. That's your cue to go into the passing lane and *walk up those steps*.

Do you play golf? Do you use a cart? If so, why? The prime physical fitness dividend from golf is not from swinging the club, which you spend very little time doing during a game. Rather, it's in the walking to the ball and to the next hole. That kind of walking is relaxing, you are almost certainly doing it with friends, and the scenery is excellent. Why pass up the opportunity to be physically active on a low-key level in pleasant surroundings? The stroll, in addition to making up for the food you may have in the clubhouse afterward, will also give you time to think about your next shot.

Tennis, anyone? There's nothing more competitive than a singles match. It's high octane when it comes to sweating off the calories and if you're up to it and in good shape, go for it. But doubles is great for its sociability element and it's just slow enough that it might get you out on the courts more often. Ideally you can work a combination of the two into your schedule.

Then there's the opportunity to take up new sports and recreational activities that will not only give you more opportunities to burn calories but also broaden your horizons. Folk and ethnic dancing will give you a good workout and probably allow you to make a whole new set of friends. Belly dancing is an ancient art that will really give you a workout. If you're short of ideas, ask friends what new activities they've tried in the last year or two.

WORK-TIME WORKOUTS

Some people have fairly substantial calorie-burning physical activity built into their workday. For example, a mailperson working on a hilly route can approach 500 calories an hour, and an emergency room doctor can hit about 230. *Fitness* magazine even calculated that Gillian Anderson burned 480 calories an hour chasing aliens on TV's *The X-Files*. But most of us lead less exciting lives and take work sitting down.

If you work in an office, you most likely have to spend most of the day in a chair. But there's still enough time between nine and five in which you could be getting a lot done while on your feet. For example, the majority of Americans use a computer for much of the day. You know that in order not to end up with eyestrain, a neck ache or backache, or carpal tunnel syndrome, you should take a five-minute break from screen and mouse every forty-five minutes or so. Why not use those minutes to take a walk in the hallway? Revitalizing your circulation will reenergize you for your work, and during the walk, you could be giving some thought to the project on which you're working.

As a matter of fact, we recommend taking an inventory of all the things you do in a typical day that could be done standing and, even better, walking. Try it next time you need to confer with someone about something important. There's something about talking and walking together that relaxes people at the same time it frees the creative flow of ideas.

Do you work in an office tower? Who says you have to take the elevator right to your floor. A great way to burn off calories is to get off two or three floors short of your floor and walk up the stairs. By doing this, you will expend extra calories, get in at least a little aerobic training where you were doing none before, and help clear your head for work.

How do you get to work? If it's close enough, consider reducing the number of wheels you use. A good walk or bike ride is a great way to start and end the workday. Leg clips will keep your good pair of pants out of harm's and dirt's way on a bike. Don't rule out in-line skates if the route is level and the weather is half decent. If you have access to a shower at work, you could even bring running shoes and shorts and take a quick run at lunchtime and then eat at your desk.

WHEN WALKING COMES WITH THE JOB

Too bad that most of us can't pick work with an eye to how physically active we will be on the job. For example, some occupations are almost as good as hiking clubs. Recently the *Detroit News* did a profile of people who ought to be wearing pedometers instead of watches. The story looked at an airlines service specialist who averaged just over forty miles in a long work week. A store manager covered twenty-eight miles, and a physical therapist, just over seventeen.

Even if your office is the open road, there's always room for a refreshing walk. Bill Kendall, a long-distance truck driver, discovered that fact somewhere along Route 80 on a trip that took him a good way across the country. Basically his activities during the trip consisted of either sitting while driving or slumped over, asleep, while his codriver was at the wheel. He also took sitting breaks at whatever roadside place served the best coffee on that 100-mile stretch. All in all, the thirty-eight-year-old Bill was beginning to display his lifestyle just above his belt, and he was not happy about it.

But now Bill is traveling lighter because he's hauling less weight on his frame. That's thanks to his dawning realization that every time they stopped in one of those huge parking lots reserved for long-distance truckers, he had a terrific opportunity to take a ten- or fifteen-minute walk around the lot. Not only did he burn calories, but he also felt more refreshed and alert when they pulled back onto the highway. Lately he's even managed to fit a little bit of skipping rope into his rest-stop workouts. (Nor does it hurt that he's also substituting whole wheat toast for the apple pie he was wolfing down with that good coffee at "Mom's"!)

CLOSING THE CIRCLE

We hope you can now see the interrelationship between all kinds of physical activity. In fact, we've just about come full circle. You've seen a broad spectrum of exercises and lesser physical activities that you can use to make sure that you burn more calories than, or at least as many as, come in with the food you eat. They range from formal exercise periods that involve routines done at specific times and in specific places, such as a gym or health club, to things we do in our everyday lives at home, at work, and during recreational time.

This most flexible of physical activities is, of course, fidgeting. It won't work miracles and you do need a commitment to begin working it into your day. The good part is that the commitment is easy, fidgeting is not terribly demanding, and over the course of time it can contribute to a better-looking you.

Fidgeting is really an extension of the general, low-level, no sweat exercise we've discussed in this chapter. Engaging in such a series of exercises is a great way to lead up to more formal workouts at the gym or at home. They rev up your muscles and joints for something bigger—not to mention put you into the right frame of mind to burn additional calories through the use of a full range of physical activities. Conversely, the more strenuous workouts make it easier for you to work more fidgeting routines into your spare time. Talk about coming full circle!

BODY MASS INDEX CHARTS

THE BODY MASS INDEX (BMI) SHOWN ON THE NEXT page is a practical marker to gauge obesity and an indicator of a more desirable weight for better health. BMI reflects a relationship between height and weight. Overweight adults (18 years or older) with a BMI ≥ 25 are at an increased risk for comorbid disease.

	HEALTHY		OVERWEIGHT			
BMI	**23**	**24**	**25**	**26**	**27**	**28**
Height	**Weight**					
5'	118	123	128	133	138	143
5'1"	122	127	132	137	143	148
5'3"	130	135	141	146	152	158
5'5"	138	144	159	156	162	168
5'7"	146	153	159	166	172	178
5'9"	155	162	169	176	182	189
5'11"	165	172	179	186	193	200
6'1"	174	182	189	197	204	212
6'3"	184	192	200	208	216	224

Height (Feet and Inches)

	5'0"	5'1"	5'2"	5'3"	5'4"	5'5"	5'6"	5'7"	5'8"	5'9"	5'10"	5'11"	6'0"	6'1"	6'2"	6'3"	6'4"
100	20	19	18	18	17	17	16	16	15	15	14	14	14	13	13	12	12
105	21	20	19	19	18	17	17	16	16	16	15	15	14	14	13	13	13
110	21	21	20	19	19	18	18	17	17	16	16	15	15	15	14	14	13
115	22	22	21	20	20	19	19	18	17	17	17	16	16	15	15	14	14
120	23	23	22	21	21	20	19	19	18	18	17	17	16	16	15	15	15
125	24	24	23	22	21	21	20	20	19	18	18	17	17	16	16	16	15
130	25	25	24	23	22	22	21	20	20	19	19	18	18	17	17	16	16
135	26	26	25	24	23	22	22	21	21	20	19	19	18	18	17	17	16
140	27	26	26	25	24	23	23	22	21	21	20	20	19	18	18	17	17
145	28	27	27	26	25	24	23	23	22	21	21	20	20	19	19	18	18
150	29	28	27	27	26	25	24	23	23	22	22	21	20	20	19	19	18
155	30	29	28	27	27	26	25	24	24	23	22	22	21	20	20	19	19
160	31	30	29	28	27	27	26	25	24	24	23	22	22	21	21	20	19
165	32	31	30	29	28	27	27	26	25	24	24	23	22	22	21	21	20
170	33	32	31	30	29	28	27	27	26	25	24	24	23	22	22	21	21
175	34	33	32	31	30	29	28	27	27	26	25	24	24	23	22	22	21
180	35	34	33	32	31	30	29	28	27	27	26	25	24	24	23	22	22
185	36	35	34	33	32	31	30	29	28	27	27	26	25	24	24	23	23
190	37	36	35	34	33	32	31	30	29	28	27	26	26	25	24	24	23
195	38	37	36	35	33	32	31	31	30	29	28	27	26	26	25	24	24
200	39	38	37	35	34	33	32	31	30	30	29	28	27	26	26	25	24
205	40	39	37	36	35	34	33	32	31	30	29	29	28	27	26	26	25
210	41	40	38	37	36	35	34	33	32	31	30	29	28	28	27	26	26
215	42	41	39	38	37	36	35	34	33	32	31	30	29	28	28	27	26
220	43	42	40	39	38	37	36	34	33	32	32	31	30	29	28	27	27
225	44	43	41	40	39	37	36	35	34	33	32	31	31	30	29	28	27
230	45	43	42	41	39	38	37	36	35	34	33	32	31	30	30	29	28
235	46	44	43	42	40	39	38	37	36	35	34	33	32	31	30	29	29
240	47	45	44	43	41	40	39	38	36	35	34	33	33	32	31	30	29
245	48	46	45	43	42	41	40	38	37	36	35	34	33	32	31	31	30
250	49	47	46	44	43	42	40	39	38	37	36	35	34	33	32	31	30

☐ Underweight ▨ Weight Appropriate ▩ Overweight ■ Obese